Post-Modern
TRIUMPHS IN LONDON

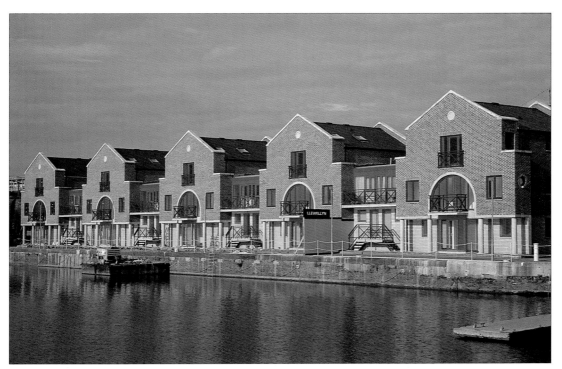

MACCORMAC JAMIESON PRICHARD & WRIGHT, HOUSING AT SHADWELL BASIN, WAPPING

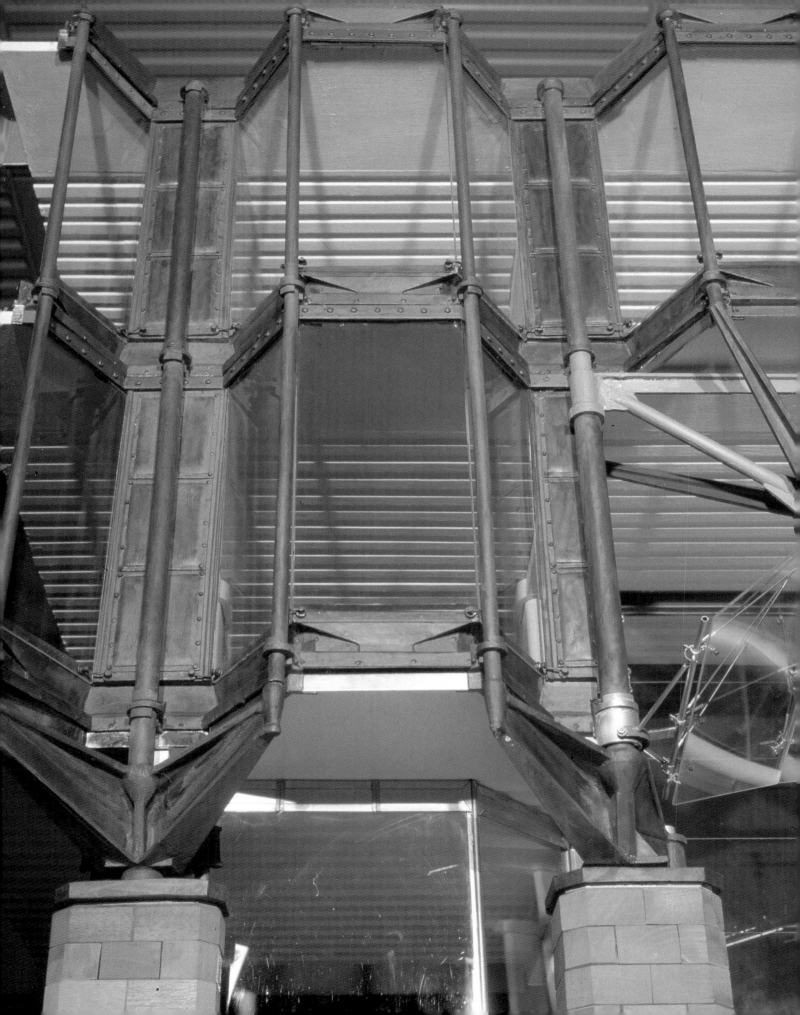

Architectural Design
Edited by Andreas C Papadakis

Post-Modern
TRIUMPHS IN LONDON

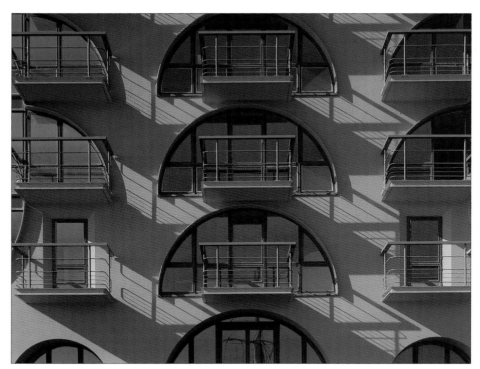

ABOVE: CZWG, CHINA WHARF, ST SAVIOUR'S DOCK
OPPOSITE: MICHAEL HOPKINS & PARTNERS, BRACKEN HOUSE, CANNON STREET, THE CITY

ACADEMY EDITIONS · LONDON

Acknowledgements

Architectural Design, several years ago, organised an exhibition and discussion on the theme of Post-Modernism and exhibited, together with an exhibition of drawings by Robert Stern, six London-based Post-Modern architects: Jeremy Dixon, Piers Gough, Terry Farrell, John Outram, James Gowan and Ed Jones. Many of the architects are now included in this choice of buildings by Charles Jencks. This issue of *Architectural Design* has been written entirely (except for the article by Kenneth Powell) by Charles Jencks. The articles and choice of architects and buildings on this occasion, therefore, do not necessarily represent the viewpoint of the Editor. *ACP*

Many of the photographs included in this profile have been taken by Justin Jencks. All other illustrations have been supplied by the architects and photographers and are credited as follows: *Front Cover* Phil Starling; *Inside Front Cover* Sheppard Robson; *Back Cover* Branson Coates Architecture; *Frontis* Michael Hopkins & Partners; *Title Page* CZWG; *National Gallery – Sainsbury Wing, An Interview pp 48-57*: *p48* Venturi Scott Brown & Associates; *p 50 below, pp 56-57* Phil Starling; *Essential Guide to 100 Buildings pp16-45, pp60-77, pp80-93*: Martin Charles *A4, A35*; Jo Reid & John Peck *A5, A8, A18, A23, A24, B22*; Richard Bryant *A7*; Dennis Gilbert *A9, B24, B25*; Jo Reid *A10*; Nigel Young *A11, A12, A12*; Richard Cheatle *A13*; Morley von Sternberg *A16*; Anita Corbin *A17*; CZWG *A19, A21*; Anita Corbin & John O'Grady *A20*; Steve Reynolds *A22*; John Outram Associates *A26, A27, A28*; Branson Coates Architecture *A30, A31*; Michael Hopkins *A34*; MacCormac Jamieson Prichard & Wright *A37, A38*; SOM *A40*; Steven Scrasse *B1*; David Quigley *B9*; Horst Kolo *B17*; Jeremy Cockayne *B18*; Mark Fiennes *B23*; Alan Williams *C2*; Leighton Gibbins *C6, C7*; Damond Lock Grabowski & Partners *C12*; Fitzroy Robinson *C17*; Ken O'Callaghan *C20*.

I would like to thank Colin Amery for identifying several Post-Modern buildings and Stephanie Williams for guiding me around the Docklands – some of her views are expressed in the captions to a few buildings there. My deepest thanks go to the many architects who have lent photographs and supplied material – particularly Terry Farrell, Piers Gough, Jeremy Dixon, John Outram, Richard MacCormac, John Melvin, James Gorst and David Quigley. Quite obviously it is their work we celebrate in this issue – an addition to the London palimpsest of another layer of history – although, undoubtedly, I have missed many other important Post-Modern buildings in my limited travels and research. *CJ*

EDITOR
Dr Andreas C Papadakis

EDITORIAL OFFICES: 42 LEINSTER GARDENS, LONDON W2 3AN TELEPHONE: 071-402 2141
CONSULTANTS: Catherine Cooke, Dennis Crompton, Terry Farrell, Kenneth Frampton, Charles Jencks,
Heinrich Klotz, Leon Krier, Robert Maxwell, Demetri Porphyrios, Colin Rowe, Derek Walker.
EDITORIAL TEAM: Maggie Toy (House Editor), James Steele (Senior Editor), Vivian Constantinopoulos, Nicola Hodges
DESIGNED BY: Andrea Bettella, Mario Bettella SUBSCRIPTIONS MANAGER: Mira Joka

First published in Great Britain in 1991 by *Architectural Design*
an imprint of the
ACADEMY GROUP LTD, 7 HOLLAND STREET, LONDON W8 4NA
ISBN: 1-85490-103-6 (UK)

Architectural Design Profile 91 is published as part of *Architectural Design* Vol 61 5-6/1991
Published in the United States of America by
ST MARTIN'S PRESS, 175 FIFTH AVENUE, NEW YORK 10010
ISBN: 0-312-06730-5 (USA)

Printed and bound in Singapore

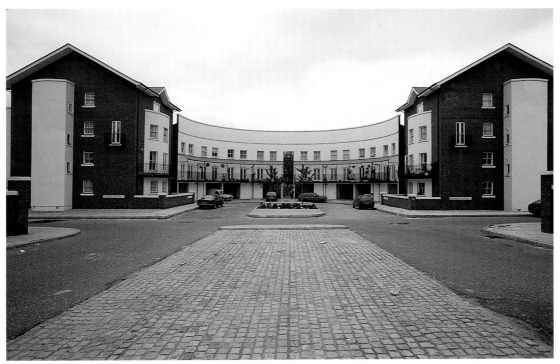

JEREMY DIXON, COMPASS POINT HOUSING, DUDGEON'S WHARF, ISLE OF DOGS

Contents
Architectural Design Profile No 91

POST-MODERN TRIUMPHS IN LONDON

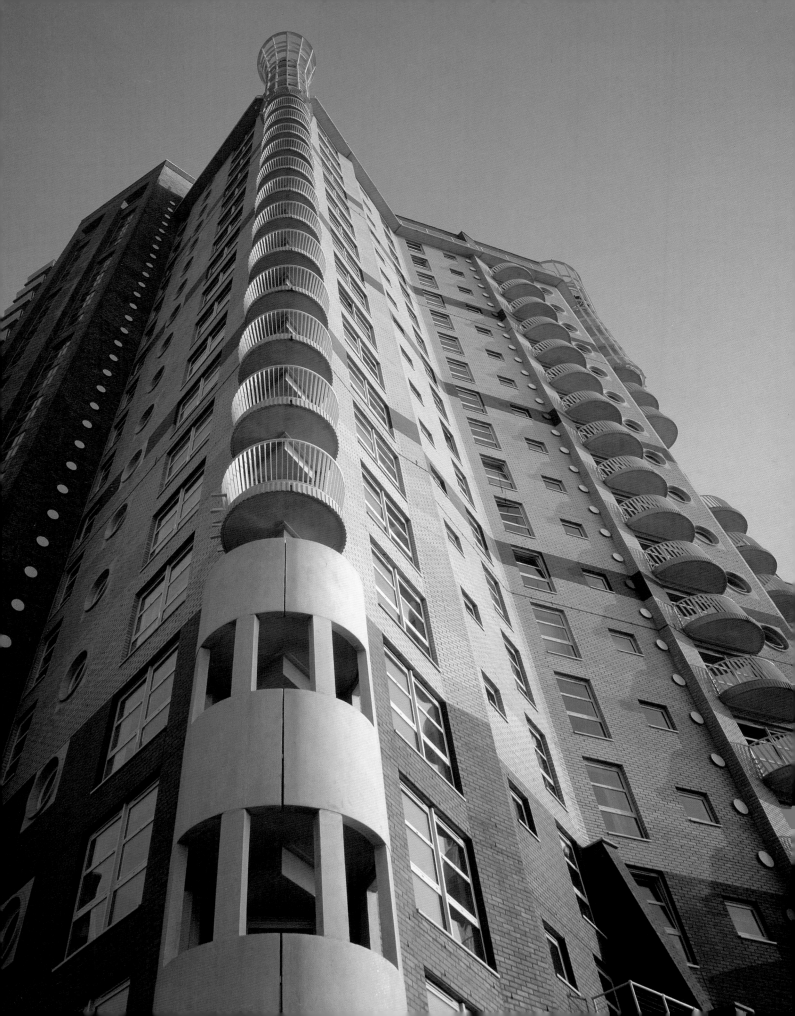

KENNETH POWELL
DIVERSITY VS DIRECTION?

My most immediate response to the decade of Post-Modern London celebrated by this issue is one of amazement at the scale and the variety of it all. I'm glad it happened – that the strait-jacket Modernist hegemony was cracked. Yet feelings of disappointment and (well, a degree of) anger follow close behind. It is too easy, of course, to brand Post-Modernism as the architecture of the Thatcher era – with all the moral and political judgements that implies. Lloyd's finished in 1986, the year that the Big Bang hit the City of London. With the Prince of Wales in a commanding position of influence and heavy pressure to please Prince, planners and public and get the buildings up, the subsequent course of events was, however, predictable. The bulk of the projects which are illustrated here have been designed and built since the mid-80s. Some are still emerging from their wrappings – looking a little lost in a world where even Terry Farrell has renounced Post-Modernism.

Farrell is the key figure, of course, and his projects markers in the development of Post-Modern London. They exemplify the true Post-Modern 'triumph': the total collapse of Modernist planning prescriptions. Embankment Place is not just a big building but the centre of a regenerated quarter. Take away the details and the building would be just as admirable. The jokes at Comyn Ching now look a bit thin, but the place is still pure pleasure. Post-Post-Modern Farrell in the 90s could be better than ever.

For the rest? Too much embodies the 'incoherence or arbitrariness of incompetent architecture . . . the precious intricacies of picturesqueness or expressionism' from which Robert Venturi dissociated himself in *Complexity and Contradiction*. There is too much that is grotesque and irredeemable – ugly and vulgar in a thoughtless way. The delicacy and the invention of the first Free Style are simply absent. There is neither consistency nor wit in, say, Chelsea Harbour.

Conversely, Post-Modernism rediscovered the street – and the good, ordinary street architecture which Rolfe Judd, Chapman Taylor, Covell Matthews Wheatley and others can do very well on occasions. Submit some of these buildings to individual analysis and they do not stand up very well. But that is hardly the point. They do not need to be judged by the standards of high art.

Of the latter quantity, alas, there is little. But perhaps there is too much of it, in a self-conscious way, in the building which some are claiming as the crowning achievement of the Post-Modern age, the Sainsbury Wing. It will function well as a place to show pictures and be popular in an unspectacular way, fading easily into the unfocused expanses of Trafalgar Square. What more can you ask? Perhaps some of the *gravitas* which is a vital quality in great architecture? Few of the millions who visit the building will appreciate the visual jokes which Jencks so relishes. Those who do will probably quickly tire of them. How many times can even a good joke be repeated before it grows stale?

In any case, London is full of Post-Modernist jokes, good and bad. Some of the best have been related by Piers Gough. None of his buildings is to be regretted but in what direction can his style develop? Has CZWG peaked? Perhaps the jokes were needed – including those of the extraordinary Ian Pollard – but the mood has changed.

The vitality – and vulgarity – of the British Post-Modernism of the 1980s is clearly rooted in the USA of Graves, Venturi and Gehry. The Post-Modern triumph in this country has not been repeated elsewhere in Europe. The contrast with France – predominantly Modernist in aesthetics and planning – brings one back to the charge that Post-Modern equals commercial/conservative/uncaring, a corollary to filthy streets and a collapsing transport system. So last-ditch Modernists struggle to save the South Bank from being Farrellised. Dirty concrete becomes a symbol of social morality, a bastion against the tide of shops.

This is ironic, since Farrell has a vision of London in which public and private again work in harmony – as they once did. Neither he nor Norman Foster, whose social criticism has become more acute of late, were willing to condemn Canary Wharf when it appeared that the much-criticised development embodied, even if in a flawed form, an inkling of that vision.

The South Bank could be the supreme Post-Modernist triumph: a gladiatorial contest with the 60s leading to a thumbs-down from the crowd and the execution of the losers. (Ironically, the architectural style of the revamped South Bank could be overwhelmingly New Modern as Farrell seeks new allies.) But perhaps the jewel in the Post-Modern crown will be Paternoster Square where the Post-Modernists flooded into the gap hacked out by the Classicists, who had to then tag along as dispirited camp followers.

At its worst, the Post-Modern triumph looks like a celebration of overdevelopment, of cynicism, of directionless disorder, of disintegration as much as discontinuity. Yet if the era is remembered with affection and respect, as well as curiosity, it will be at a time when the diversity of London was both rediscovered and reinforced. For all the horrors, that is no mean achievement.

Kenneth Powell is Correspondent for The Daily Telegraph, *and member of the Academy Forum Council.*

CZWG, Cascades, Isle of Dogs.

DECEMBER 1990

British
TELECOM

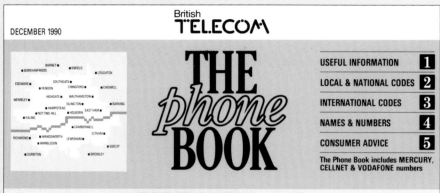

THE
phone
BOOK

USEFUL INFORMATION	**1**
LOCAL & NATIONAL CODES	**2**
INTERNATIONAL CODES	**3**
NAMES & NUMBERS	**4**
CONSUMER ADVICE	**5**

The Phone Book includes MERCURY,
CELLNET & VODAFONE numbers

RESIDENTIAL L-Z

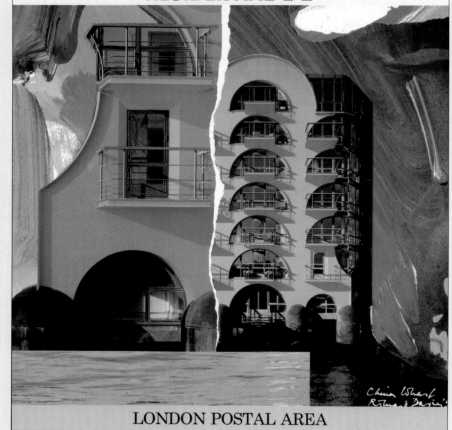

China Wharf
Rilwyn & Davies

LONDON POSTAL AREA

CHARLES JENCKS
POST-MODERN TRIUMPHS IN LONDON

In the last ten years the texture of London life has changed dramatically. The transport system and infrastructure have declined, London Docklands has been turned into a kind of Houston Texas, the City has been Big Banged by mega-buildings – four million square feet of new office space in the boom years – and a host of Post-Modern flowers, and weeds, have sprouted up in every quarter. This issue of *Architectural Design* shows the dissemination of a world movement in one city – it is a guide to, and critique of, what is now an ubiquitous approach. But can this sudden influx of a foreign plant be called a 'triumph'? And what would victory be – or defeat for that matter?

Capitalism is said by Robert Heilbroner, among other eminent economists, to have triumphed over Socialism in the last three years, and we know what a hollow conquest that has been. In 11 years of governmental asset-stripping Margaret Thatcher only managed to lower State spending from 43 to 38 percent of national product – a pyrrhic victory – and the proportion has started to climb back up again. Capitalism, a totally free market unregulated by government and devoid of monopoly influence has not, and never will, exist. How, then, could it possibly triumph?

Warfare

While triumph may also be questionable in the architectural world, no one can dispute that conflict has reigned in the past decade. The vocabulary of critics is that of the battlefield: a 'victory' for Modernism is proclaimed in Paris with the opening of IM Pei's pyramid; a 'setback' for Traditionalists is announced when Prince Charles has to trim his Dorcester plans; Post-Modernists 'suffer another defeat' when Michael Graves' Whitney extension is axed for the third time, and New Modernists achieve a 'clear win' when Bernard Tschumi and his team of Deconstructionists are given the *carte blanche et rouge* at the Parc de la Villette.

Battle, warfare, defeats and victories are inherent in the politics of architecture, as they are in other discourses. The world of art politics is also beginning to resemble that contested territory seen by Michel Foucault as the basic ground on which we live and struggle. Is it a Darwinian battlefield? For him, power was both decentralised in individuals – literally in bodies – as well as centralised in such structures as the judiciary and the state, and this led him to the idea that war was a permanent condition, and metaphor, for thought, as he said in an interview 'Truth and Power', 1977:

> Isn't power simply a form of warlike domination? Shouldn't one therefore conceive all problems of power in terms of relations of war? Isn't power a generalised war which assumes at particular moments the forms of peace and the State? Peace would then be a form of war, and the State a means of waging it.

Or again:

> One's point of reference should not be to the great model of language (*langue*) and signs, but to that of war and battle. The history which bears and determines us has the form of war rather than that of a language: relations of power, not relations of meaning. History has no meaning . . .

Yet for Foucault history had the meaning that power-discourse reveals the struggle between individuals, groups and nation-states. Language uncovers this struggle and embellishes it with all sorts of epigrams. Think of the barbed metaphors that Prince Charles has hurled against Modernists, calling their buildings 'a monstrous carbuncle', 'an academy for the secret police', 'a nuclear power station' or Post-Modernist work, 'an old 1930s wireless' (2). Think of the contemptuous dismissals of the opposition one hears every day in the political realm – or even within a party during the Heseltine-Thatcher 'battle'. Not only do brutish metaphors dominate – nasty militaristic or animalistic figures of speech – but words of combat, crushing and killing. If, with the Deconstructionists, peace is really war by other means, today so venomous are the epithets flying through the media, so palpable the intolerance, one has the impression that if words could kill, humanoids would recently have become extinct. What kind of 'triumph' could there be for Post-Modernists in this situation?

Holy War

Since his Mansion House speech three years ago, Prince Charles has been steering his 'crusade' away from the Modernists and directing it at Post-Modernists. Perhaps sensing at last that the former had already been vanquished, some 15 years earlier by the latter, he shortened his reins, snapped down his visor, waved to the troops massed behind him – Classicists, Ecologists and assorted Establishmentarians – and charged straight at Sir Philip Dowson and his winning scheme for the Paternoster area.

An honourable knight of the realm was skewered by a Prince armed to the teeth with media power and backed by BBC polls. These supporting forces, raised from the shires, were used to clout Sir Philip into submission. Not content with abusing his scheme verbally – as a 'spiky prison camp' and 'half-hearted watered-down Classicism' – the Prince orchestrated a switch to the John Simpson counter-scheme by inviting the new developers to Highgrove, where they dutifully picked his choice and dumped the competition winner. How prescient of them! They had little choice, given the *de facto* power the Prince had demonstrated in stopping or stalling five major London schemes.

Perhaps sensing that he was going a bit far, the Prince pulled in his lance when he addressed the American Institute of Architects (AIA) meeting in Washington DC in February 1990, and merely tilted playfully at a few Post-Modernists, mocking their 'signature buildings' and damning their 'stonework pared down to the thinnest sheets modern technology can produce'. While attacking this 'wrapping paper' architecture out of one side of his visor,

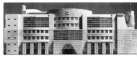

1 *Post-Modernism goes public – CZWG's China Wharf (A23) has been used, like other London PM buildings, as a telephone book cover by British Telecom.*

2 *James Stirling & Michael Wilford, Number One Poultry, London EC3, 1989. Not an 'old 1930s wireless' but a well-scaled Post-Modern Classicist building, with V-windows, banded courses and many other hallmarks of the style which happen, also, to be contextual to this part of the City of London.*

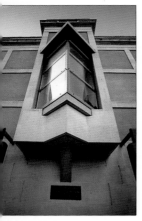

3 *James Stirling & Michael Wilford, Clore Gallery, Tate Gallery Addition, 1982. The V-windows became ubiquitous in London after this building was finished.*

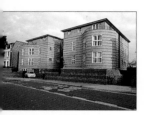

4 *Pollard, Thomas & Edwards, Goldhawk House, Goldhawk Road, 1988. Banded brick courses and Rossian windows – Post-Modern vernacular.*

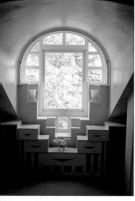

5 *Charles Jencks and Terry Farrell, Thematic House, 1979-85. The curve and stagger – 'face' and 'tree' – Serliana and Jencksiana.*

he congratulated one of the dreaded enemy, Kohn Pedersen Fox, out of the other, and handed them an AIA award.

Here is one of the ironies of his Holy War: while continuing to tilt at windmills tagged 'Mod' or 'Po-Mo', he has seen this just redoubles their strength and number. Here they rise up at the RIBA in the form of an adolescent President and a whole generation of 'Neo-Mods'; there they sprout all over London where most firms are now building in the Post-Modern style. The Prince has even seen his cherished Paternoster area subtly infiltrated by Post-Modernists like Thomas Beeby and Terry Farrell. And if built to the Neo-Classical specifications Prince Charles supports, it will be a clip-on revivalism, the thinnest form of wrapping paper possible because that is what economics plus technology allows: a steel frame with a two-inch facade. It will be counterfeit as Classicism *and* deceitful as Post-Modernism. Can that be considered a 'triumph' for either side?

For more than ten years the RIBA (the Royal Institute of British Modernism) has been leading its counter-crusade against 'Rats, Posts and other Pests' as Aldo van Eyck so charitably called them in his Discourse of 1981. 'Hound them down, let the foxes go' he urged to the cheering, jeering audience of blood-lusting Mods on the rampage. Berthold Lubetkin, Bruno Zevi and other Old Modernists soon followed and a yearly, sometimes monthly, bloodletting occurred within this professional establishment. It's true, of course, that during Rod Hackney's presidency blood flowed the other way and, for a time, Modernists suffered the same kind of summary judgement from Community Architects (and even Prince Charles, who was allowed into the enemy camp). But this was only a brief interlude. The ritual slaying of the Modernists gave them just enough impetus to regroup for a counter-attack and mount a campaign under the banner of President 'Mad Max', as he is affectionately known. He established his credentials, of course, with a book attacking the Prince. Michel Foucault would not be surprised at any of this.

Architectural warfare has become so endemic that Modernists and Classicists ritually abuse each other now by accident, a consequence of the linguistic syndrome they have constructed. Both sides demonise the other like political opponents, both groups justify their own 'Fascist' tactics with stories of the other's despicable behaviour. As with the Palestinians and Jews both parties are convinced that the injustices they perpetrate are justified by those of the others. Point to an undemocratic act of Prince Charles and Leon Krier will remind you of the 50-year suppression of Classical architects; mention the illicit awarding of prizes, positions and commissions to Modernists and they will tell you how Traditionalists all but control the shires, the countryside.

At the debate on the Prince's *Vision of Britain* exhibition at the Victoria & Albert Museum in 1989, carnage reached a new level of mindless ferocity as Martin Pawley compared Prince Charles to Pol Pot, then Leon Krier likened a Modernist to Honecker; then Sandy Wilson compared Prince Charles to Hitler; then Lucinda Lambton compared a Modernist to Ceaucescu; then Martin Pawley compared Prince Charles to Hitler . . . if words could kill!

Desire

Of course the building debate is a little more civilised than that in Northern Ireland and a real architectural murder has not occurred since Stanford White was shot in New York more than 80 years ago (and that was a lovers' quarrel). No, architects are cultivated people and they spend most of their passionate time – that is, the few hours devoted to feeling – focused on the things they love, the creation of new form languages, architectural ideas, moves in the great game of urbanism. Here, as Foucault would remind us, is another source of power, a positive individual one, perhaps as strong as the coercive and destructive power of warfare.

Desire, creativity, sexuality – all these life forces have generative power which can quite overwhelm the negative or repressive brand. Note how Post-Modernism swept through the architectural world when the movement was at its most creative, from 1977 to 1985. There was nothing the Modernists or any other group in control of the Establishment (the AIA, the RIBA, the academies) could do about it. Insults, taboos, zoning laws, academic purges had little effect. If anything the attacks of the Aldo van Eycks merely fanned the flames of illicit desire and spread the passion further. Or think of how the New-Modernism stole the blush of youth from the aging Post-Modernists and by 1988, with the Deconstruction Show at MoMA, had come to epitomise virility, glamour – in a word, desire. All the forces which society tries to contain, or redirect to social ends, are liberated in architecture when a new formal language comes into being. Could this be the triumph of Post-Modernism in London?

Undoubtedly by the middle 1970s a whole gamut of new forms which looked fresh and untried were presenting a challenge. The creative potency of the unexploited new idea can be compared to the excitement felt by miners striking an entirely new vein of ore. Almost nothing can stop architects, certainly architectural students, from immediately tapping this fresh source. And so we find the sudden outbreaks of a new fashion for strange uses, something that looks irrational to those not under its spell. What were the forms that sparked the Post-Modern explosion? There were three obvious sources, the three main form-givers. In the 60s, the skewed and complex spatial ideas of Robert Venturi; in the 70s, the stripped Classicism and square windows of Aldo Rossi, and in the early 80s the Cubist Classicism of Michael Graves. In addition there was a new form language which came from anonymous sources. Collectively those formulae have established the very identifiable Post-Modern style in London. What are its salient characteristics?

Walk down any major street now, or look at the photographs here, and you will inevitably discover some recurrent details. Two window types are so ubiquitous as to be clichés: the small, square cross-mullioned Rossian window (B7) and the V-shaped protruding window (3). Why have these solutions turned up everywhere? Ask a psychohistorian and you may be told their symmetries indicate a return to a body-centred language, a form that at once frames the view and holds the viewer. Ask James Stirling about the prow-shaped windows at the Tate and he will say they provide a sudden view of the garden and a 'penetration' of the exterior by the interior space, a break in the skin. Or perhaps they simply give a more original way of lighting to the enclosed gallery space inside. The proliferation of a new formal device obviously has both functional and psychological causes.

There are some forms whose arrival is more purely ornamental. The sudden acceptance of banded masonry is a good example of this more gratuitous fashion (4). Why should vernacular housing now always come in courses of banded brick? (B8, B18, B21) Architects say it is to break down the mass, and obviously it also accelerates the vertical tempo of a structure and lessens its regularity. The justification more generally is 'Why not?' – it's playful, colourful, relatively unusual and just as cheap as a monolithic brick facade. But architects are always searching for a deeper justification – a relation to underlying structure, or the surrounding context, or the internal symbolism of the building.

One formal solution that I have reused 30 different ways in the Thematic House – the curve and stagger – is now also frequently found on the top and bottom of City buildings, such as those at Broadgate or One American Square (5, 6). This form-type resembles many natural things, including a face and the tree: the top curve isn't at once the forehead or crown of leaves, the bottom rectangle can be a nose, neck or branched trunk depending on how it is articulated. It has the advantage of combining opposites – curved and straight lines, gentle undulation and sharp staggers, masculine and feminine. It can also be stretched in other dimensions, like the Serliana motif, to help the designer surmount formal problems such as inconsistent bay rhythms or left-over space. Terry Farrell has used it in TV-AM (A7), Embankment Place (A11) and Alban Gate (A13) to give an anthropomorphic presence to a facade. His skyscrapers reach up to their 'heads', while his hovering beetle of a building at Charing Cross suppresses its 'forehead' below its shoulders (7). But the anthropomorphism is mostly subliminal and that is its strength. It merges with the architectural context – other arches and staggers – and thus can sink below the threshold of recognition, not always being a 'face' or a 'tree'.

Most of the buildings in the City of London have adopted the general Free-Style Classicism which is the hallmark of Post-Modernism as a public language. It has become something of a businessman's vernacular for the same reason the International Style did 30 years before. Whereas that language was abstract, rational, no-nonsense and thus an appropriate style for daily work – the equivalent of the pin-striped suit – Post-Modern Classicism is suitable as the entrepreneurial mode. Yuppies dressed for their boardroom conquests are clothed in an outer skin of pink granite which is polished, or flamed within an inch of its depth. Modernists such as Deyan Sudjic or Jonathan Glancey – or Prince Charles for that matter – love to hate this 'wallpaper' and find it phoney and pretentious (which it often is).

But they miss the major point: architecture has always had a symbolic role, long before the Greeks represented their wooden temples in stone, and the Modern Movement, Le Corbusier no less, justified the potential liberated by skeletal construction as 'the free facade'. Modernism brought in the two-inch 'curtain wall' – have these critics perhaps forgotten? – and it is as natural to our way of life as the two-piece suit. Every businessman now wears this, from Peking to Sao Paulo, just as every business centre now makes use of the steel frame and clip-on facade. The reasons are technical and economic. 12-inch stone facades are too heavy and expensive; besides, it is only the surface we ever see. The Romans knew this when they clad their great brick baths with a stone veneer, or even worse from a puritanical viewpoint, stuccoed and painted the brick structure to resemble stone.

Perhaps some critics would dismiss the lessons of Greece, Rome and Le Corbusier, but some Post-Modern architects such as Arups have devised interesting ways of translating them into the present. At Broadgate, for instance, Peter Foggo has designed the curtain-wall as a hung masonry grid, turned the stone on its side to show it

as veneer, and extended it sharply from the actual glass skin to show its non-structural capacity (8). Here is typical Post-Modern truth, its characteristic detail. Stemming from Stirling's demonstration of structure and cladding at Stuttgart, Foggo has *constructed* an ornamental layer of flamed and polished masonry and featured it as construction. The two-inch block is here turned sideways to the building to create at once a sunshade and demonstration of snap-together detailing. The patterns of contrasting small bronze clips, black voids and masonry are a pleasure to behold, forming a surface which proclaims its non-functional role, its separation from enclosure.

If the non-load bearing facade is expressed as clipped, then it is also expressed as layered. Layering is a characteristic Post-Modern motif that results naturally from constructional necessity and, again, cost. If one wants the light and shadow of a traditional stone – the 'empathetic architecture' of Michelangelo and Geoffrey Scott – then it must today be created either in the cast stone methods developed furthest by Ricardo Bofill, or the flat, layered method of most Post-Modernists. This latter system results from placing one thin layer of construction on another – steel, wood, concrete, stucco, and overlapping them at an edge so a series of shadow lines result. Lansdowne House in Berkeley Square is a commercial version of the layered facade (9), Jeremy Dixon's Housing in St Marks Road a more thoughtful example (A3); but low- or high-minded, they all make a virtue of faceting. The results can resemble the fractured surfaces of Cubist architecture in Prague, which also expressed planes of material superimposed as layers.

One could continue enumerating the particular qualities of Post-Modernism, the motifs, stylistic formulae and urban ideas. There are 20 or more that make it a coherent language, which I discuss in subsequent sections: the urban perimeter block, the new terrace housing, the urban piggy-back building, the new industrial Baroque style, asymmetrical symmetry and so forth. All these ideas, methods and forms were new enough in the early 80s to stimulate architects and clients into action. For a while they created the erogenous zones of architecture, pockets of desire and mystery which were more powerful than any possible censorship. Now they constitute the texture of more than 100 buildings in London and have created whole areas of the City such as Broadgate. But with this consummation has also come a loss of desire. Acceptance leads to familiarity, vulgarisation, mass-production – can this cheapening be the triumph of Post-Modernism?

Modernism Improved
Perhaps its most indisputable improvement on Modernism has been with the slab block – especially where this has been refitted, refurbished, repainted or completely transformed. There are many 1960s buildings in London with concrete frames and a dour grimace which have been given a Post-Modern face-lift, and in virtually all the cases the cosmetic surgery represents an improvement in terms of skin tone, colouring and cheerfulness (C18, C19, C20). It is hard to think how it could be otherwise. The cheap 'rent-slabs' of this period were a kind of degree-zero of expression (it is interesting that Modernist critics such as Bruno Zevi today even propose a 'degree-zero aesthetic' to ward off the dangers of Post-Modern rouge). Most people hate these former megaliths: 'the grey, empty, obtuse stupidities in which we live and work will bear humiliating evidence to posterity of the spiritual abyss into which our

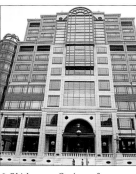

6 *Skidmore, Owings & Merrill, Broadgate Development, Bishopsgate Road, 1987-91. The body/ face motif returns three times to give a human scale to 12 storeys.*

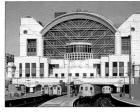

7 *Terry Farrell Partnership, Embankment Place, Charing Cross, 1987-90. The 'head' is lowered between two 'shoulders'.*

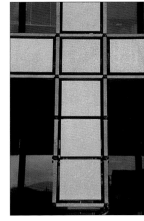

8 *Peter Foggo and Arup Associates, Broadgate Development, 1988. Post-Modern detail features its clipped-together role as the new ornament through the black shadow lines, the clips and the polished and matt masonry.*

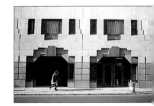

9 *Chapman Taylor, Lansdowne House, 1987-88 – the layered, fractured skin.*

11

generation has slid' (the words are Walter Gropius', 1919, but they apply perfectly to these office gravestones).

Most of the Post-Modern refurbishments go beyond cosmetics and transform the acoustics, space, grammar, air-conditioning, function, view, entrance lobby – and just leave the underlying concrete or steel frame. One of the better examples is Sheppard Robson's 338 Euston Road, a 16-storey office block which now has a strong Classical bone structure (which is the air-conditioning), an elegant curving forehead and a crisp, ivory-coloured skin (10). In terms of function, interior comfort and beauty this is a clear improvement on its Modernist predecessor – who says there isn't progress in the arts (Vitruvius believed there was?)? The alternative method of renewal – blowing up – is crude. Post-Modernisation can be just that: the modernisation of Modernism. There are enough examples in London and Glasgow of 'before and after buildings' to convert even the greatest sceptic to the posterior movement. The RIBA should conduct re-educational tours of these improvements.

New Cultural Logic
In all discussions of the movement – in literature, sociology, film – Post-Modernism is always seen as displacing the Modernist distinction between high and low culture. Instead of being élitist it is pluralist; rather than being limited to an avant-garde or educated coterie, it also seeks out the market-place and populace (1). The characteristic double-coding of the style is based on this truth: it must appeal to both high and low taste cultures. Even more, it should cut across a spectrum of castes and if not unite a fragmenting culture – an impossible task – at least appeal in different ways to different people, or the same person in various moods. Polymorphism, multivalence, pluralism: these are its key words.

To see how distinctive this position is, one only has to contrast it with the other prevailing theories of culture. Whereas Prince Charles attempts to reimpose an integrated Classical culture – *du haut en bas* – or his opposite Stephen Bayley in his show on *Taste*, 1983, attempts to legislate a Modernist integrated culture – *du bas en haut*, Post-Modernists search for variety, opposition and difference, *en haut, en bas, et au milieu*. They believe that a field of opposites creates meaning, that taste is not, as Bailey or Prince Charles believe, good taste alone, but wide, various tastes. Think of the difference between Racine and Shakespeare, or Corelli and Mozart. The latter of both pairs understood that real taste was eclectic – the inclusion of bad, mediocre and refined taste in a field of tensions. Shakespeare and Mozart did not repress difference, otherness or even vulgarity – instead these became personified elements in their dramas, characters which provided social realism and wit.

In literary criticism, especially that Post-Modern variety stemming from Mikhail Bakhtin, such opinions are commonplace. As he argued, the heteroglotic tradition of the novel, building on the polyphonic work of Rabelais and Cervantes, reaches one culmination in the 19th century with the novels of Dostoevsky. According to Bakhtin, this Russian writer allowed various voices to interact in his novels without suppression, without imposing his single, authorial voice. Since then this 'dialogic' (for polyphony is most open in the dialogue) has deepened, and the Post-Modern novels of Umberto Eco, David Lodge and John Barth are the sites where different languages converge, where opposite ideologies play. They are no more inte-

grated than James Stirling's addition to the Staatsgalerie in Stuttgart – the epitome of eclectic confrontation, where four different codes of architecture achieve parity. This polyphony, David Lodge and others point out, resembles that of the carnival.

The architectural parallels are quite obvious. Think of the work of Piers Gough, or John Outram, or Ian Pollard (A16-25, A26-29, C1-2): it may differ in quality and intention, but it is all polyphonic. Ian Pollard will mime the languages of James Stirling at Stuttgart and then turn them into farce and commerce (11). Low-Cult has always borrowed from High-Cult, and in this case the borrowing is doubly ironic since the lender, Stirling, originally borrowed some of his coinage from the high street. In this double borrowing who has lost credit, or – as the pun would ask – has Stirling been devalued? No one would mistake Pollard's Homebase for a serious essay in eclecticism, there are too many quotation-marks in the references, too many obvious jokes, indeed, like a carnival, too many obvious everythings.

The carnival, however, is a serious manifestation of city pluralism, a celebration of difference and the end of distinct categories. In the annual Notting Hill carnival (13) a riot of 'otherness' is channelled between buildings, contained by the police, but nevertheless allowed to break out in visual expression. Blacks, social outcasts, youth, tourists, voyeurs, those from the neighbourhood, dogs, police horses, women on floats, students, businessmen in disguise, rent-collectors, old-age pensioners, indeed all social types mingle and jostle in the spectacle. In a carnival categories and class distinctions don't matter. Pastiche and the transgression of boundaries triumph for a moment; there is a holiday from rationalisation, a day-off from classification. Beggars become performers, dolls become queens, reggae and exhibitionism mock the pretension of social stability.

The Post-Modern carnival of building in London curiously occupies the centre of society and power – that is the City of London. It is here one will find the most outrageous pastiche, and liberation from the usual binds of good taste and breeding. Here, driven no doubt by the profit-motive and the market notion of value ('the difference that makes a difference') are located the palaces which mime ancient Rome and Florence, but with such a brazen falsity that no one could take them for the real thing (C11, C12, C13, C15). Pomposity, Classicism, hierarchy, authority, the past – most of Prince Charles' rules of good architecture – are confirmed, and then parodied, either knowingly or unintentionally (12).

No one will mistake such buildings for their High-Cult counterparts, because the clip-on facades are so thin and so caricatured. These are not counterfeits, as they are accused of being, not even a child would be fooled. No, they are pragmatic parodies, no-nonsense fantasies, inexpensive variations on grand themes. They may be damned for being shameless about their opportunism, but their deceit is nonetheless straightforward. Commerce has always played this slightly subversive role: it looks for a cheaper way to send new messages, to manufacture information, to create 'the difference that makes a difference'. The definition of information, as formulated by communication engineers, confirms this truth of the marketplace. Information in a product always tells the buyer what is different, what distinguishes it from every other choice on the market. For this reason a city, a marketplace, is *the* mechanism for sustaining difference.

It is no accident then that Post-Modernism has triumphed

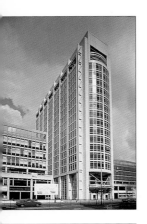

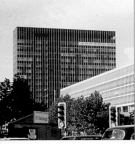

10A & B, 'Before and After' refurbishment of a 60s office block, Sheppard Robson, 338 Euston Road, 1989-90. A PM Order of elegant steel columns holds the services, extends the former space 1.5 metres and provides acoustic and climatic control not available in the original slab block.

as a commercial style right in the heart of the global marketplace. As a mode or language it mixes new and old, ideal and real, in acceptable measure. Commercial Classicism used to do this, especially when it was Art Deco, but Modernism never really tried. Tied to a 'monologic', as literary critics might say, it never took in the diversity of city life, its very real carnival. By contrast, the Free-Style Classicism that Michael Graves forged in the early 1980s became the international heteroglot of all commercial centres around the world. One America Square as well as Farrell's City buildings are constructed in this style, a language which will accept new technology, strange urban sites, new and old buildings, Blacks, youth, tourists, rent collectors . . .

Heteroglossia is the new cultural logic as Bakhtin, Lodge and Eco make clear, the polyphony that allows 'difference' to emerge and takes its place alongside the 'dominant'. This eclecticism does not mean the Post-Modern architect has to give up his own distinct language, or lose her identity in the mélange of languages, any more than the Post-Modern writer loses an authorial voice. Rather, as these critics and writers argue, the author's particular point of view remains as one more among many – a privileged but not totally determining role, an organising but not reductive function. In Post-Modern novels, *Small World*, *The Name of the Rose*, the author may appear, disappear, try to dictate and try to listen – but many voices and genres are always heard. There is a theme and a certain unity of plot and discourse, but essentially difference prevails.

This, to answer what has now become a rather rhetorical question of this essay, is the 'triumph of Post-Modernism in London': the emergence, celebration and containment of difference. Whereas triumphs of architecture in the past concern the adoption of a single Classical or Modern Style, the victory for Post-Modernism – accidental though it may be – is that five styles now coexist, on relatively equal footing. It is the only architectural party which can win if, and only if, its opponents also can claim victory. New cultural logic indeed. Neo-Modernism dominates the young, Late-Modernism rules much of the profession, Revivalism reigns over Prince Charles, vernacular also wins in the shires and Post-Modernism leads commerce: together, all five approaches establish a system of difference and, if society can sustain that difference over the years, it will be more than a rhetorical 'triumph' for Post-Modernism. Its pluralist goal will have been given foundations and become more than the happy accident of a collision between commerce, confusion and a swarm of angry monists. For the pluralism today is more the fortuitous by-product of competing, power-driven zealots than it is the conscious creation of tolerant bystanders. No architectural constitution, or proportional representation, guarantees that it will last. Prince Charles may not be Hitler, Modernists may not be Honeckers, but if the work of any of them depended on the tolerance of the other, it wouldn't last more than a season.

Thus Post-Modern London means a diverse and contradictory city and an architecture I have here, somewhat arbitrarily, divided into three sections – A, B and C – canonic buildings, urbane buildings and those that typify the carnival. The architecture will not be to everyone's liking, and occasionally I prefer 'bad' to 'good' buildings. My intention in writing the captions and placing the architecture is less to judge than to demonstrate heteroglossia, less to give opinion than to uncover what has happened in ten years. The diverse architects whose work is shown here constitute something of a hidden tradition, an unconscious club, a cryptic brotherhood and if, in showing their buildings, they and the public begin to appreciate this emergent school, then this guide will have served its purpose.

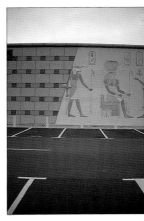

12 *Renton Howard Wood Levin Partnership, One American Square, 1989-91. Post-Modern Classicism as the knowing commercial style, one part parody, one part pragmatism.*

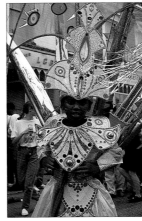

11 *Ian Pollard, Sainsbury Homebase, 1988, uses several of Stirling's Stuttgart styles and slides them into Egypt and a parking lot, marking the differences, as here, with ironic signs.*

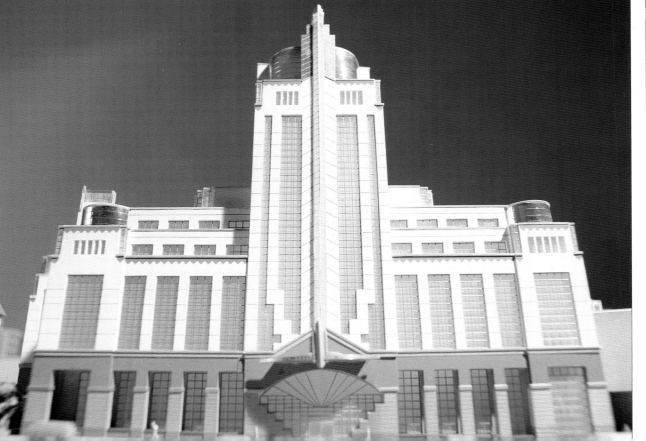

13 *Notting Hill Annual Carnival, 1990.*

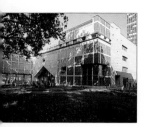

The Chameleon – Stirling and Wilford's Clore Gallery changes its skin five times in this view, and twice more around the next two corners. There are now quite a few Pop versions of this genre (see C1 and C22).

Can one speak of a 'London School' of architects? Is there an identifiable group of Post-Modern architects at work, comparable to the 'London School' of artists, a group which shares assumptions and a related style? Only where one finds common paradigms – that set of problems, and ways of doing things that establish canons.

Post-Modernists in London, like creators elsewhere extending and deflecting a tradition, are engaged in an argument with previous design solutions. As Harold Bloom has shown in *The Anxiety of Influence*, poets may swerve away from the very models they seek to emulate. They do this to achieve a psychic distance from their chosen exemplars, to carve out a space of freedom from old rules and habitual solutions; at the same time they reassert respect for the tradition they subvert. This double process, a form of benevolent hypocrisy, produces a development later identifiable by the historian as a 'sequence', the story of history. But the contemporary critic may also be able to identify imminently growing sequences, in effect the canons of which the poets and artists are only dimly aware. For Post-Modern architects in London, as elsewhere, the canons of the new urbanism have become, by the 1990s, quite explicit.

Most familiar of these emergent rules is the *perimeter block*, the row of buildings (usually housing) which extend around a city block holding the street lines while ringing the changes on whatever motifs and organisational types are at hand – adjacent window patterns, cornice lines and rhythmical proportions. Good examples of the perimeter block are Jeremy Dixon's housing at Compass Point (A5), CZWG's Sutton Square (A19) and Orchard Mews (A21). The last two create enclosed U-shaped space on the inside of the block, and a contextual wall full of incident on the outside. The formula is the basis of the old London Square and Parisian *place*, and it has been taken up by virtually all the major Post-Modernists – for instance Richard MacCormac at Shadwell Basin (A35) and a host of followers (see examples A33, B9). CZWG is more calculating than most other architects in swerving hard from the model – thus making it fresher – by adding such non-London flourishes as corner towers and warped scroll mouldings of gargantuan size.

In London many other Post-Modern formulae are used which are also internationally shared: the *infill block*: Terry Farrell's Comyn Ching (A10); the *piggy-back building* (both Farrell's Air Rights Building at Charing Cross and John Outram's Blackfriars building, (A29); the *wall building* which, for instance ties two street lines together (B21); and the *positive figural void* (almost all of CZWG's urban work). For instance, their recently completed The Circle creates a very strong figural void in plan which is then played with and distorted in elevation. Dark blue, almost purple, glazed bricks around an absolute circle are punctuated by diagonally placed balconies and 'owl ears' (or 'vase lips' as Piers Gough prefers) (A25). The pure geometrical figure is thus counteracted, softened and bent by two other strong figures – an obvious 'swerve' from the precedent.

The most distinctively new urban canon is the *chameleon building*, a model unique to Post-Modernists because only they really stress pluralism and eclecticism – the variety in expression which flows from the coexistence of many different cultures. The essence of any contemporary city today is the simultaneous presence of different orders: different ethnic groups, different taste cultures, different clusters of consumers, different classes, different professions. Difference is recognised at all levels of Post-Modernism, by writers, philosophers and artists, but it is perhaps urbanists who have to deal with it most directly because the city manufactures fast-changing and splintering taste. Only in the urban realm are variety and the conflict of world views finally guaranteed and protected. People lose tolerance the further one moves from the city centre – although, of course, today it is a polycentre. This has resulted in a different kind of architecture.

Whereas previous ages may have produced schizophrenic oppositions – the Classical front versus the Queen Anne behind – whereas Alberti changed sex and mood from female refinement to brutish vernacular as he went around the corner of the Palazzo Rucellai, no architect before the present switched skin colour and tone four or five times depending on the surrounding context. This shows our new-found respect for difference *per se*, for history as both rupture and continuity.

The most advanced versions of the genre are Stirling and Wilford's Clore Gallery (A1), Jeremy Dixon and BDP's Royal Opera House Extension (A6) and Robert Venturi's National Gallery Addition (A2). All three change style to suit the adjacent buildings, or those across the street; all three change mode at unusual points in the facade (not just the corners); and all signal a change in relative value of functions with a shift in material so that entrances and ceremonial spaces are more highly ornamented than sides and behinds. It all looks very odd, because it is so different from Modernist and Classical canons of articulation. Needless to say it is rejected by these traditionalists.

At the Clore (A1) Stirling adopts six styles which sometimes slam, or knit, into each other as they wrap around the circuitous site; at the Royal Opera House (A6) Dixon uses about four modes, and at the National Gallery (A2) Venturi *et al* have employed five (if one counts the re-entrant glass courtyard). These numbers indicate how seriously the Post-Modernist takes difference; but they also suggest a latent conflict with the normal rules of integration, something about which I questioned James Stirling:

Charles Jencks: Some, Traditionalists particularly but also Modernists, will feel the building contrasts too much with the old Tate.

James Stirling: I don't think so and the real situation was that we had to get the building through several types of approval. I felt that deferences had to be made to the existing Tate and connections, like stone courses and parapet heights, and materials like Portland stone had to be repeated. So the building comes out from the side of the Tate, turns round a corner and comes in behind the lodge – which I thought should be preserved as it maintains a symmetrical balance with a similar building on the other side of the Tate. But as the new building moves away from the Tate it becomes different and more eccentric and begins to express its own personality.

CJ: Well, I think it's a chameleon building fitting into several different environments which for me is very exciting and a new idea, taking contextualism to a new level. I mean you've joined up the parts, not on the edges where other architects would have done it, but sometimes a quarter way down the facade and then you've overlapped them too. A Classicist or a 19th-century eclectic architect would change style at the corners and make a front and back . . .

JS: I don't think you can make junctions on corners because if you do, the transition is too strong – it becomes a break . . .

In further answers Stirling stressed the need for continuity, smooth transitions rather than abrupt cuts, thus underlining a paradox: while differences can be underplayed by elision, they can also be heightened if they appear side by side for comparison. Difference *and* continuity are both sought here and in the Post-Modern paradigm generally, an opposition which underscores the fact that pluralism *and* co-operation must coexist to make either one possible.

While the chameleon is sometimes considered the most opportunistic and devious of animals, these realists show that buildings following its lead can deal with the deepest problems of varying function and differing world view. Pluralism finds its expression and most fitting emblem in this quixotic animal. Of all places it is London where the changeable organism has emerged and in this sense one can say it defines a 'London School'. Are other urban cultures more conformist?

The Perimeter Block – but surrounding a square of water – Richard Reid Architects, Finland Quay West (A33).

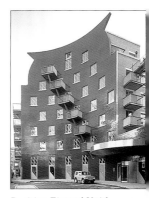

Positive Figural Void – CZWG's The Circle (A25) encloses a circular space and reinforces this shape with the curious 'owl ears' or 'vase lips'.

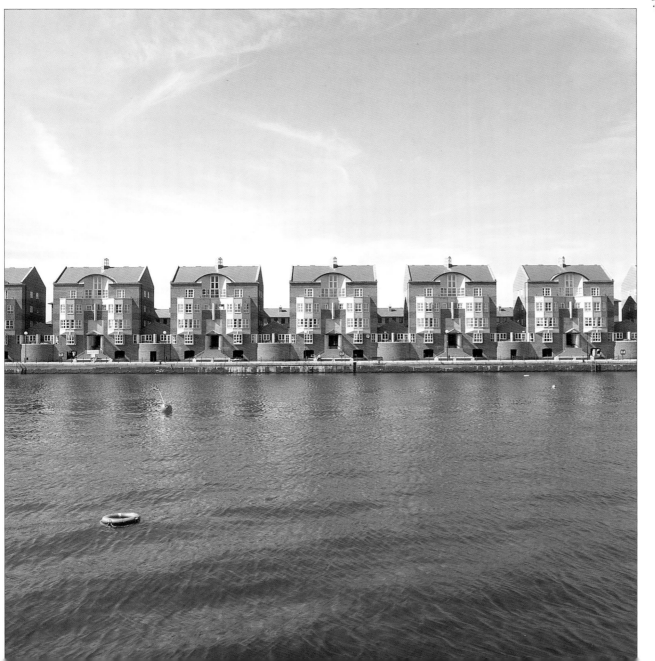

43 CANONIC POST-MODERN BUILDINGS

A1 *JAMES STIRLING & MICHAEL WILFORD, Clore Gallery, Tate Gallery, Millbank SW1, 1982-86. Six styles knit and slam their way around the site in perhaps the greatest game of contextualism played to date. Sometimes a detail is borrowed directly from the Old Tate – the cornice – sometimes it is subtly inverted – the pediment and semicircular window over the entrance. Occasionally the adjacent brick building is referenced, or at the back, the utilitarian role of the building. An architecture for all seasons which, when the garden grows and the trellises are full, will nestle in comfortably to its mixed context.*

A2 *VENTURI SCOTT BROWN & ASSOCIATES, Sainsbury Wing, National Gallery Addition, Trafalgar Square WC2, 1987-91. London, indeed English, Classicism reinterpreted by the Italian-American Robert Venturi. The sequence is a* tour de force *of sliding and interpenetrating themes. Like Stirling at the Tate, Venturi borrows the cornice and a few pilasters and columns from the older museum, then he staggers them densely in a Baroque manner as 'ghosts'. This theme ends with a crescendo of columns and a final coda: one almost free-standing Corinthian. Here a heavy black void also marks the entrance, along with a few sectioned mouldings, and the grammar suddenly slides into a style that might be called Portland Stone Renaissance. But it has black Miesian inserts! From there it melts again into a flat wall expanse and – Stirling-like – changes texture and mood after it turns the corner on Whitcomb Street.*

Here it is 'Dickensian London' – stone base, stock yellow brick and modern gallery lights. Finally, around the corner, this street vernacular is broken by the sign 'The National Gallery' and given a sweet Classical surround. English Classicism always has such idiosyncratic mixtures, Venturi argues, and so the chameleon exterior changes yet again at the top – as Nash would do – to show the actual function, the gallery lighting. Such contrasts are realistic and expressive: the grand interior stairway, the elliptical connecting bridge and the well-scaled galleries are excellent – Post-Modernism at its doubly-coded best. More wilful are the Egyptian capitals (why, if one is going to design symbolic columns, not a 'British Order'?). And the culmination of the heroic stairway is a banal elevator. Nevertheless, this is the most accomplished pluralist building in London.

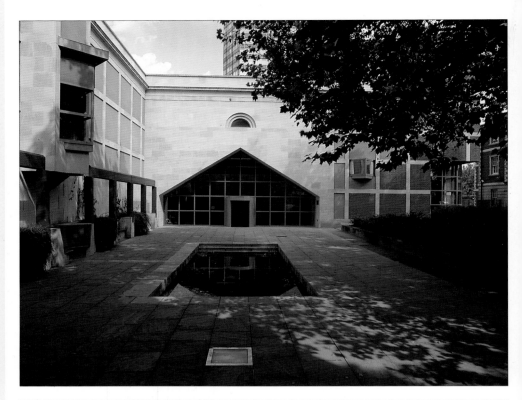

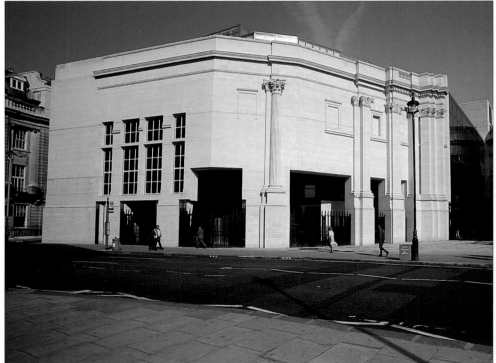

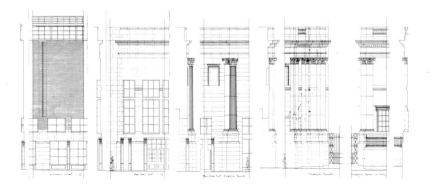

A3 JEREMY DIXON, St Marks Road Housing, North Kensington W11, 1976-79. Sophisticated and complex Post-Modern Classicism that isn't all it seems: three houses are tucked into the single house form and backs are shifted at an angle to the front facade because of the angled site. An anthropomorphic visage is hinted at, as are pyramids, De Stijl and crow-stepped gables (with the gables upside-down). This scheme was, for its time, the Post-Modern answer to inhuman Modernist slab blocks.

A4 JEREMY DIXON, Housing, Lanark Road, W9, 1986. Flats treated as villas raised high above the automobiles. Dixon achieves a dignity with minimum means – dark brick, cream render, deep eaves of a Tuscan persuasion, syncopated stairways and arched windows. The basic decisions are sensible and powerful: hold the street line, tower above the cars, and put semi-private areas at the back.

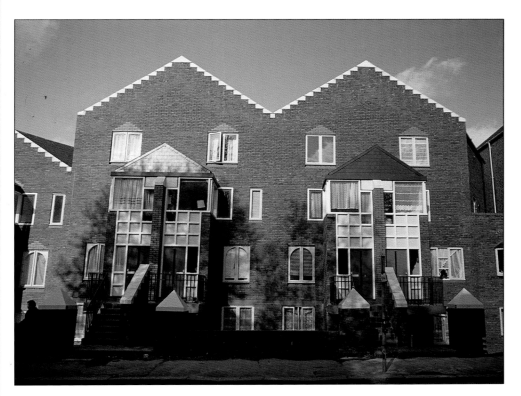

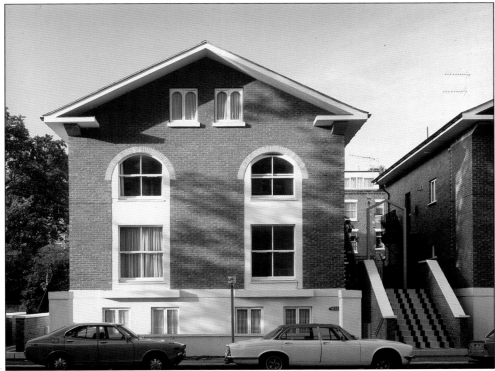

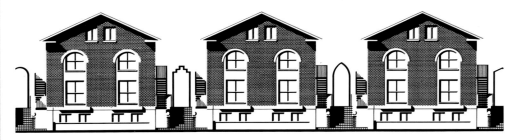

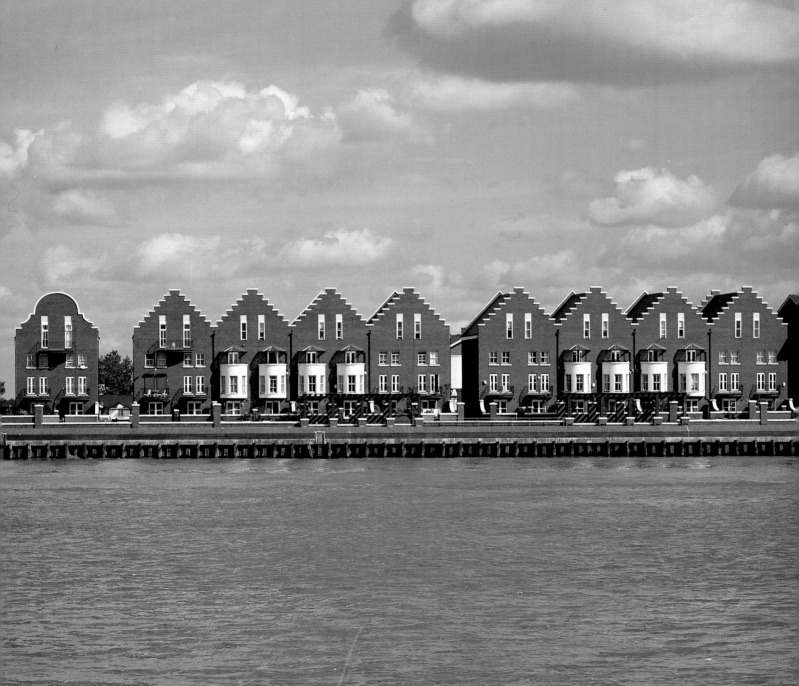

A5 *JEREMY DIXON, Compass Point Housing, Dudgeon's Wharf, Isle of Dogs E14, 1988.* 152 flats and houses organised according to three London typologies: as terrace housing along the river front, as a broad avenue of semi-detached villas in the middle and as cheaper courtyard housing at the back. Transition points are marked by higher buildings, towers in the grammar Dixon has adopted. Dark brick and light render unify the three typologies and, for the most part, distinguish between main surface (brick) and protrusion or setback (render). The English-Dutch gables add slight articulations. This unity in variety makes it the most urbane and civilised set piece in the Docklands. No other housing approaches it for the basic urbanistic decisions: a sheltered river walkway with pergolas and seating areas versus a dignified avenue culminating in a modest 'circus'. The villa typology creates a very nice rhythmical balance between architecture, automobile and entryway – that is between the ideal and the all too real.

A6 *JEREMY DIXON + BDP, Royal Opera House Project, Covent Garden WC2, 1987-90.* A chameleon building fitting into four different environments: 18th-century London stonework on the piazza side; Post-Modern Classical on commercial Russell Street; rehabilitated engineering next to the Opera; and informal vernacular on the roofscape. Modern horizontal windows and traditional pergolas are quoted directly – as are the rectangular voids from the Uffizi placed above the arcades – but these quotes are sensible and not overbearing. They give just the right amount of figural presence to Dixon's background grammar. The interior also continues the mixed grammar of recognisable elements set in a new contextual background.
Painting by Carl Laubin specially commissioned by Architectural Design *for the publication of* Post-Modernism and Discontinuity *featuring* L to R, *Andreas Papadakis, James Stirling, James Gowan, Leon Krier, Charles Jencks, Terry Farrell and Fenella Dixon.*

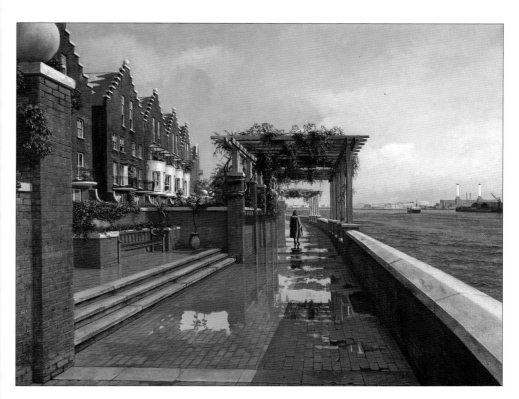

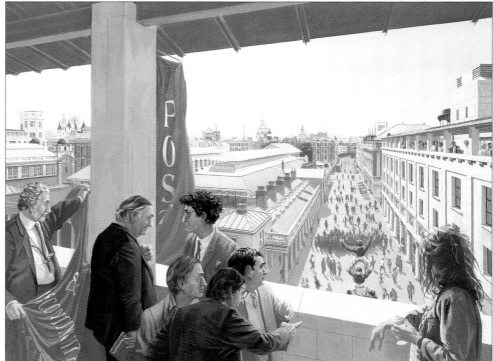

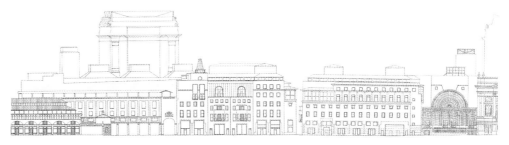

A7 TERRY FARRELL PARTNERSHIP, TV-AM Breakfast Television Centre, Horley Crescent, Camden Town NW1, 1981-82. The first of Farrell's bottom-heavy buildings which accentuates the rise to the top through various formal methods. Here this acceleration is achieved by the Renaissance palazzo device of increasing the speed of rhythms as each floor surmounts the next, becomes smaller and slightly steps back. To say the extruded letters, TV-AM, are exaggerated is an understatement. Most symbolic images are emphasised – the steel-frame keystone (for entrance), the eggcup finials (for breakfast TV) and the interior garden landscape (for civilisation) – but as an inexpensive conversion that captures the symbolism of its evanescent media role, this confection can't be beaten.

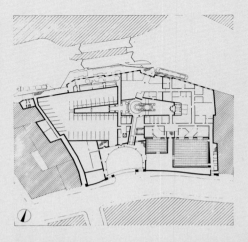

A8 TERRY FARRELL PARTNERSHIP, Midland Bank, 95-97 Fenchurch Street EC3, 1983-87. Banking hall and offices. A contextualist building that turns a triangular corner nicely, with a customary tripartite elevation that abstracts the detail as it rises. Note the bolted ornament.

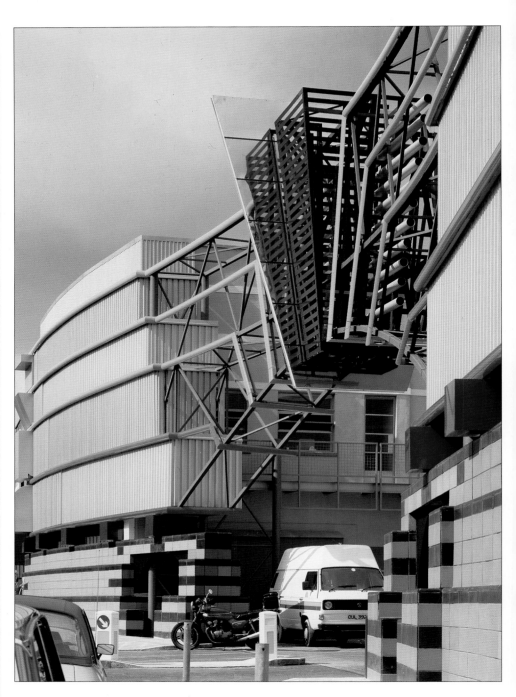

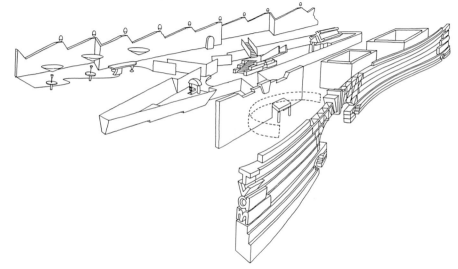

20

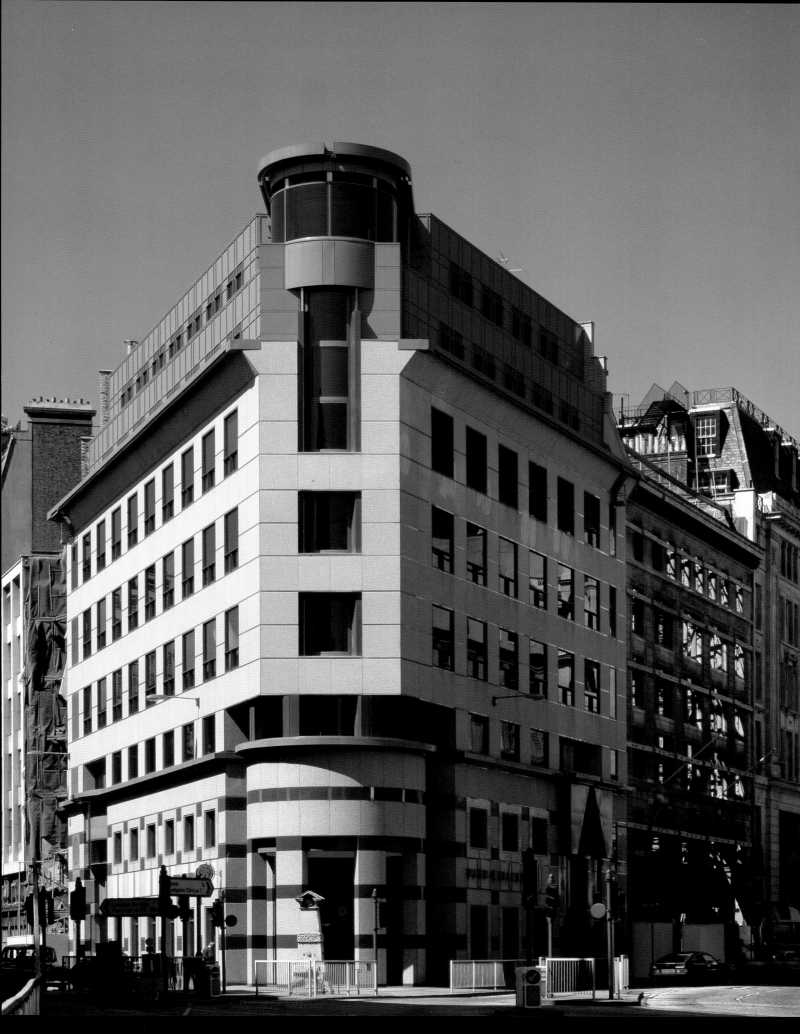

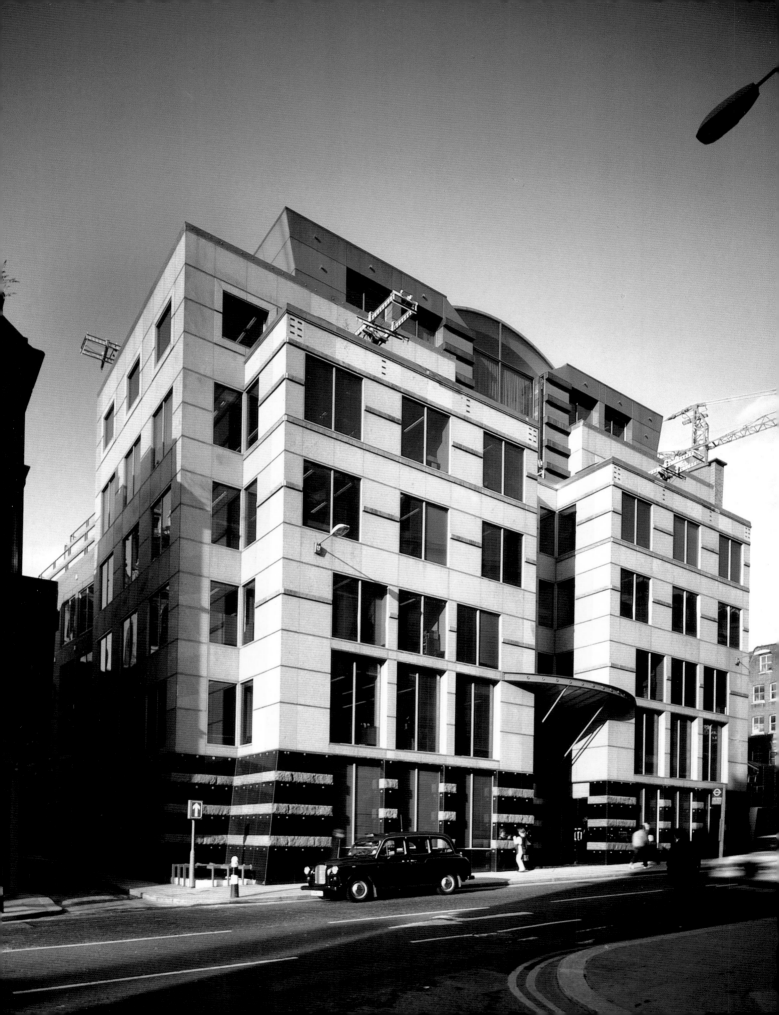

A9 TERRY FARRELL PARTNERSHIP, Allied Irish Bank, Queen Street EC4, 1982-88. Office and bank development. Symmetrical office building with exaggerated bolt-ornament emphasising that all the panels are clipped to a steel frame. This Post-Modern Classicism stems from Otto Wagner's Secession Building, but is given an unexpected twist through the stepping back and diminution of forms rising from an ultra-heavy base.

A10 TERRY FARRELL PARTNERSHIP, Comyn Ching Triangle, 19 Shelton Street, Covent Garden WC2, 1979-90. Mixed development of offices, flats and shops, both converted and newly designed. The interior courtyard is the most effective part with Lutyensesque tricks played by the entryway that turn the viewer into the triangular enclosure. There one discovers coved and sectioned mouldings stepping up the slope in a syncopated manner mixing Baroque and Mackintoshian flavours.

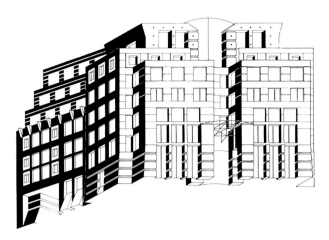

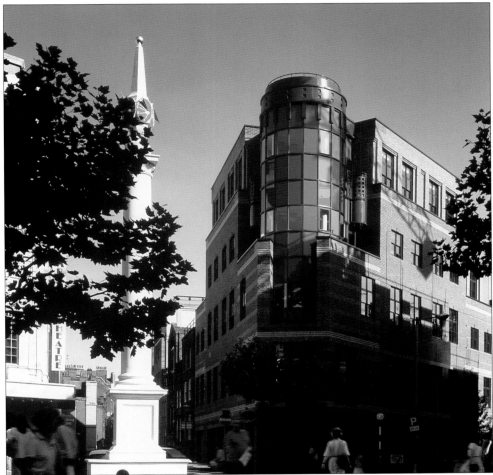

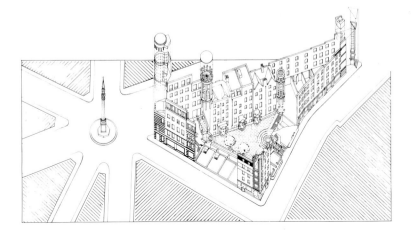

A11 TERRY FARRELL PARTNERSHIP, Embankment Place, Charing Cross WC2, 1987-90. A heavy beetle crawling across the London skyline? Heads which have collapsed between two shoulders? Characteristically, Farrell uses a Gravesian Post-Modern Classical grammar, but accentuates the weight of the building, like an Edwardian architect. Partly this is just financial sense — more activity near the ground — but the aesthetic of stepped-back, diminished arches runs through many schemes. The contrasts of heavy and ultra-thin steel tension members, solid and void, could not be more extreme. At the base, where the trains enter, wonderfully squat columns inflect both to the colour of British Rail and the industrial/Classical aesthetic. Their extruded sections have a powerful sculptural quality that contrasts with the more fastidious lighting elements that punctuate the platforms.

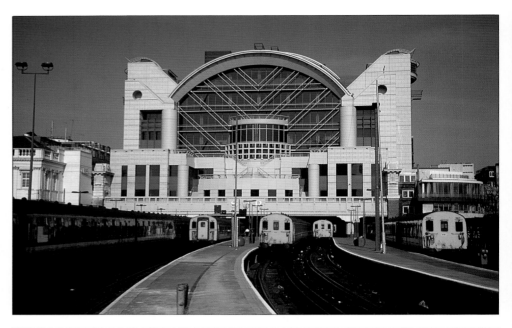

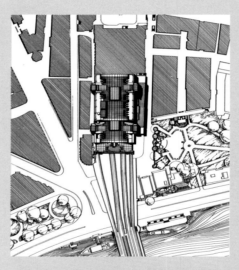

A12 TERRY FARRELL PARTNERSHIP, Tobacco Dock, Pennington Street E1, 1989. A six-bayed warehouse conversion of an 1804 building into shopping village on two levels. The original mixture of timber and early cast-iron technology is by Farrell's 'interventions' of staircases, industrial balustrades and an original version of the Doric. All this is compatible, straightforward and suitable to the new entertainment functions.

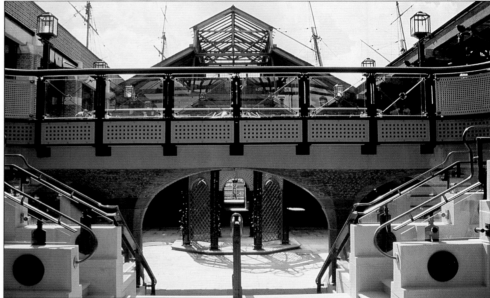

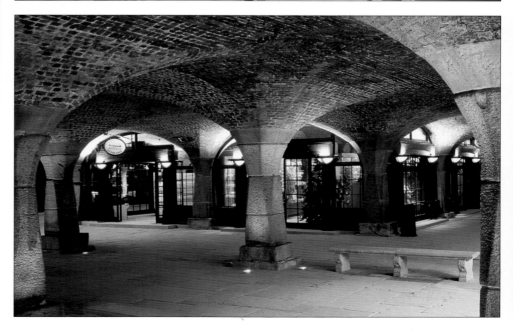

A13 TERRY FARRELL PARTNERSHIP, Alban Gate, London Wall EC2, 1987-91. A major office development spanning London Wall. Two bottom-heavy towers are set skewed to each other like lovers having a quarrel. The articulations do break the scale but, regrettably because of planning interventions, the facades have been coarsened and the two 'heads' diminished.

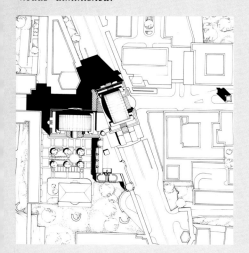

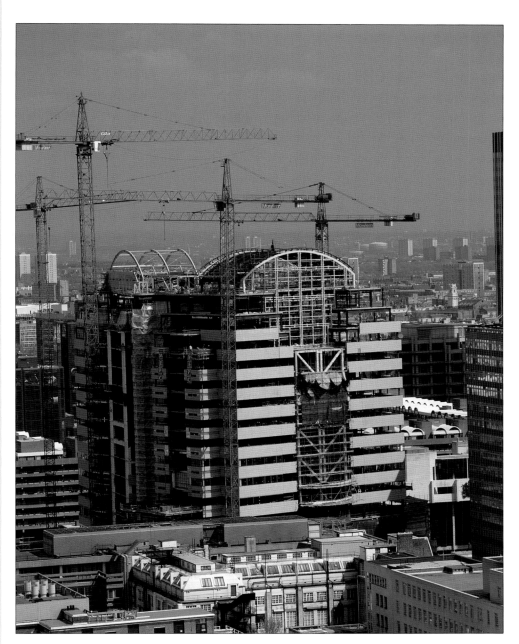

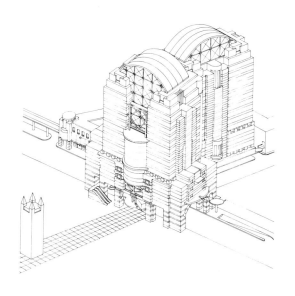

A14 TERRY FARRELL PARTNERSHIP, *Vauxhall Cross, 80-85 Albert Embankment SE1, 1989-92.* Over 400,000 sq ft of offices with car park, new riverside wall and walkway. The office as a hanging garden makes a spectacular use of the riverfront views. Farrell's work on other Thames 'palaces' has paid off here in this imaginative way of breaking down the massive office into a series of interlocking terraces. The result may be a cross between Hollywood, Graves, Bofill, Mayan ziggurats, Art Deco and Beaux-Arts planning, but who said Post-Modernism is pure? Very convincing is the handling of the rhythms, of foreground to background, solid to void, stone to glass. Note the way the ziggurat of masonry syncopates into the glass pyramid – a pleasing beat set against a calm absolute symmetry.

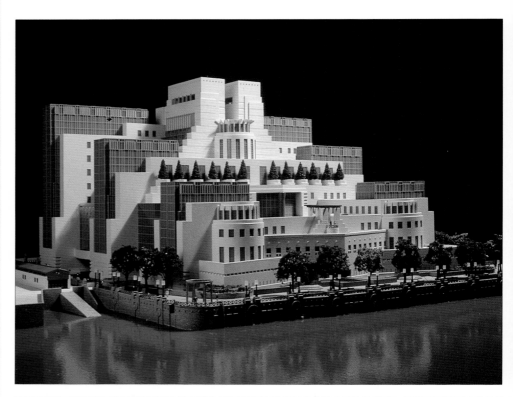

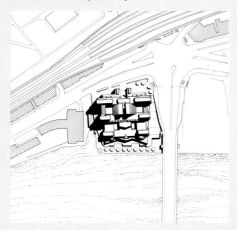

A15 CHARLES JENCKS AND TERRY FARRELL, *Thematic House, Holland Park W11, 1979-85.* Two heads, or 'Jencksiana', on the street side and four with bodies on the garden side are the main ordering devices of these two facades meant to bring an anthropomorphic and symbolic role back to architecture.

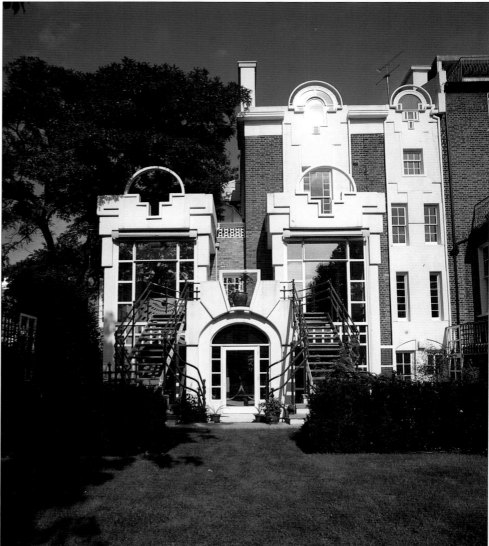

A16 *CZWG, Phillips West 2, 10 Salem Road, Bayswater W2, 1975-76. The new West London headquarters for the auctioneers, this transformation of a warehouse combines auction rooms, offices and residential space. The architects claim it as London's first Post-Modern building because its brick structure was painted pink and then 'loaded up' with symbolic and expressive features: pantile roofs, pyramid tank rooms, arched parapets and bolted-on steelwork for balconies and entrance canopy give a variety of rhythms.*

A17 *CZWG, 33-35 Gresse Street, Fitzrovia W1, 1982-83. Inspired warehouse conversion created the first purpose-built designer studio in what has now become a 'designer enclave'. A solid London yellow brick factory building with concrete lintels has been given a new facade centred on a pair of huge two-storey circular windows.*

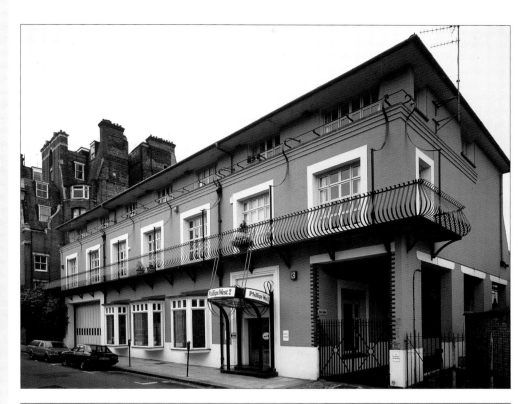

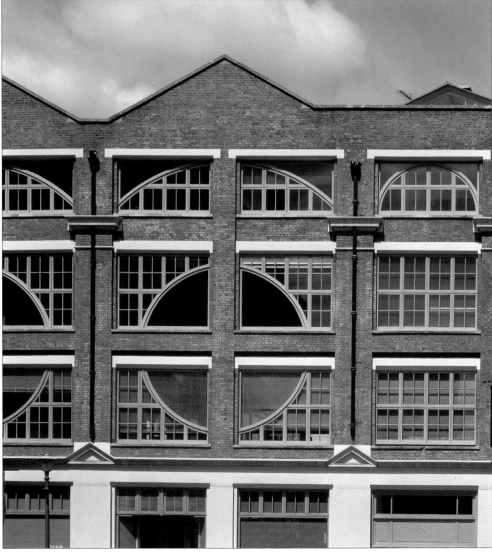

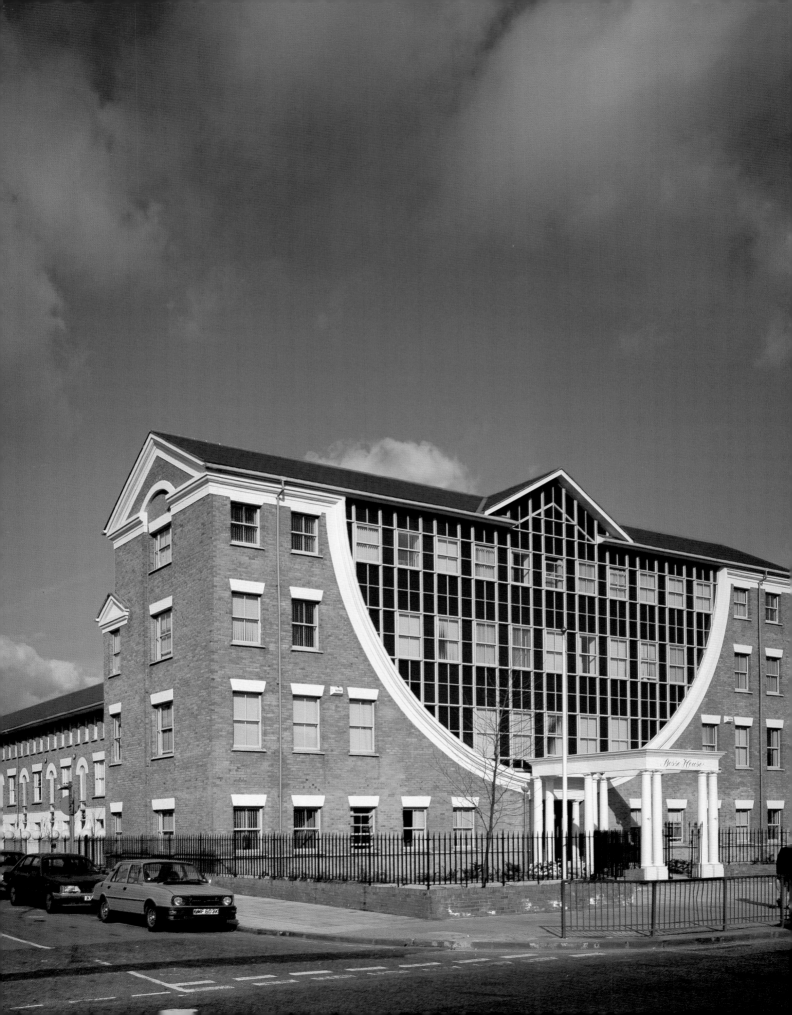

A18 *CZWG, Besso House and Eaton Terrace, Mile End Road E1, 1983-85. CZWG describes Besso House as inadvertently Mannerist, and 'probably the thinnest office building in London', a modest office block with an assertive Ledouxish facade featuring a highly decorative, functionally useless entrance pergola. But this idea of clothing an office with developer's Georgian and then peeling it back with a huge moulding and upside-down arch makes it the supreme example of Post-Modern wit in London, a humorous conceit used to reveal the truth.*

A19 *CZWG, Sutton Square, Hackney E9, 1983-85. Created from a former industrial site backing onto a church, this intimate square provides 49 houses and 16 flats in a commercial development. The architects have reinterpreted the traditional terrace housing with street-front and garden-back, and given it some Lutyensesque touches and strange proportions: here the Dutch scroll gable is expanded, and their white stucco forms are turned upside-down.*

A20 *CZWG, Royalty Studios, Ladbroke Grove W11, 1984-86. Brick-built development for spec-built designer-workplaces, carried out on a tight budget. The ghosted, circular window details are similar to CZWG's Gresse Street facade and have become a popular motif for other conversions in the area. Ever since Robert Venturi used steel 'ghosted figures' in 1972, it has been a hallmark of Post-Modern design.*

A21 *CZWG, Orchard Mews, De Beauvoir Town N1, 1986. Half-acre residential development on a former industrial site in a 19th-century neighbourhood, the mews groups 15 timber-frame and yellow stock brick houses around a small courtyard. Four corner 'sentinel houses' are given turret bedrooms, clad in terracotta tile and crowned with aluminium cupolas reminiscent of Lutyens' New Delhi Chatris. The asymmetrically placed cornice windows remind one that, in spite of the straight revivalism, the architects still consider themselves* Post-Modern.

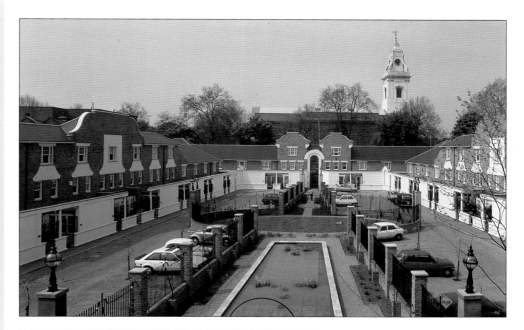

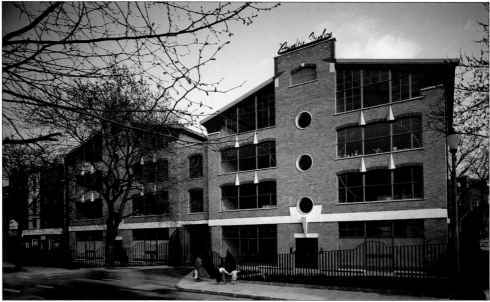

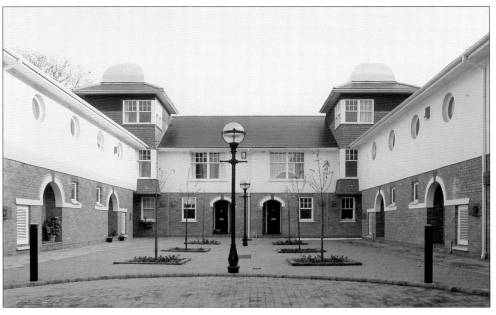

A22 *CZWG, Janet Street-Porter's House, 44 Briton St, Smithfield EC1, 1986-87. An idiosyncratic home-office using four colours of brick which graduate upwards from dark to light in the Gaudian manner. The chaos is more apparent than real because many elements – windows, some balconies and open screens – are ordered geometrically into huge diamond patterns. The variety of room shapes is suggested by this collision of diamonds.*

A23 *CZWG, China Wharf, 29 Mill Street, Tower Bridge, Bermondsey SE1, 1987-89. This development of flats and offices was built to fill a hole in the line of waterfront wharfs, wedged tightly between New Concordia (to the right) and Reed Wharfs (left). It shares a lift and entrance with these two behind a surprising white-faced scalloped wall which is meant to recall industrial silos nearby. Characteristically the architects have turned the recollection inside out, just as on their red-arched front they have played games with pagodas, ships and the ubiquitous 'wharfism' of the Docklands.*

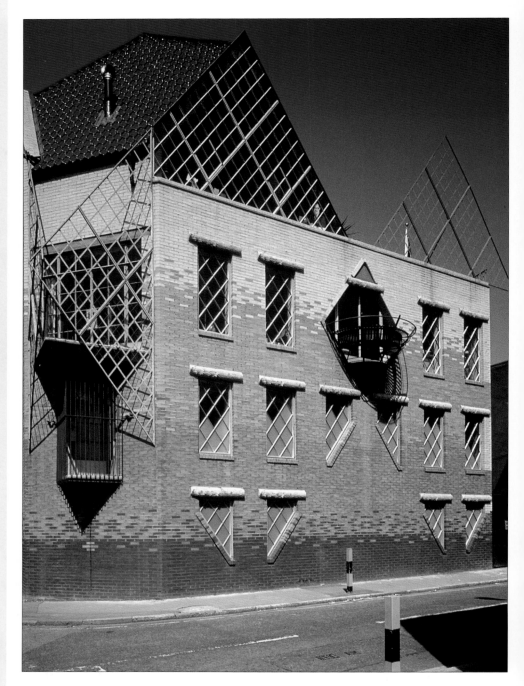

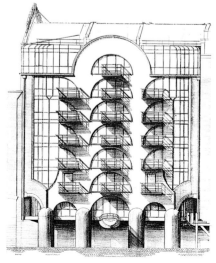

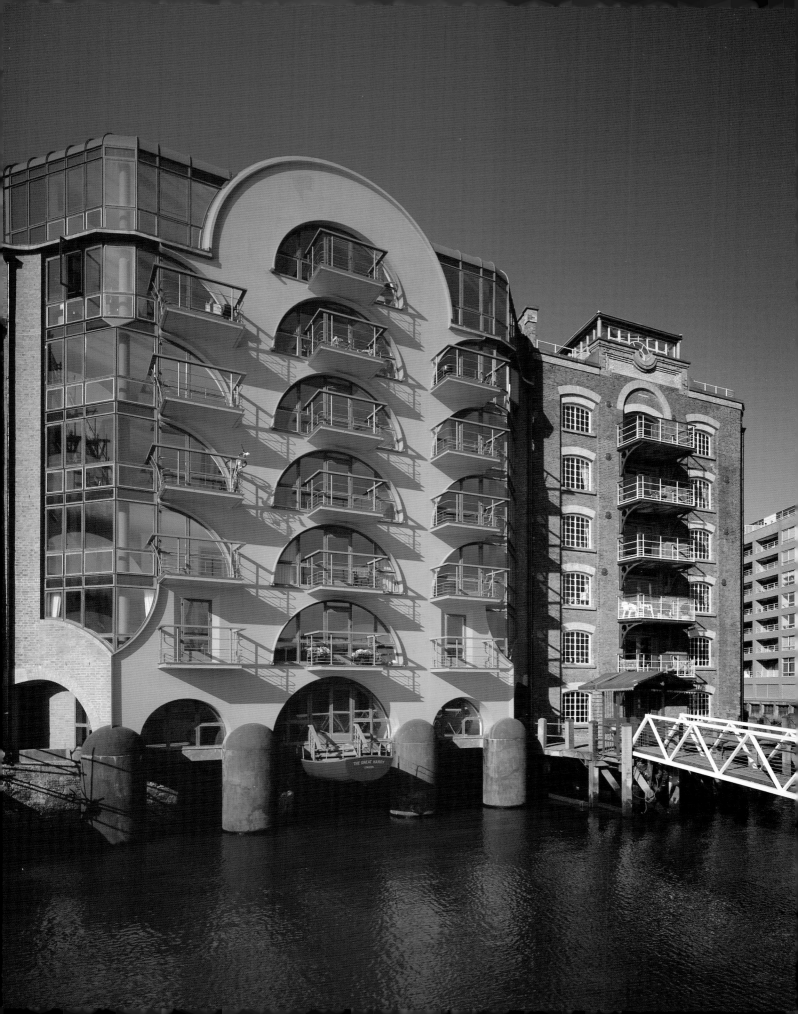

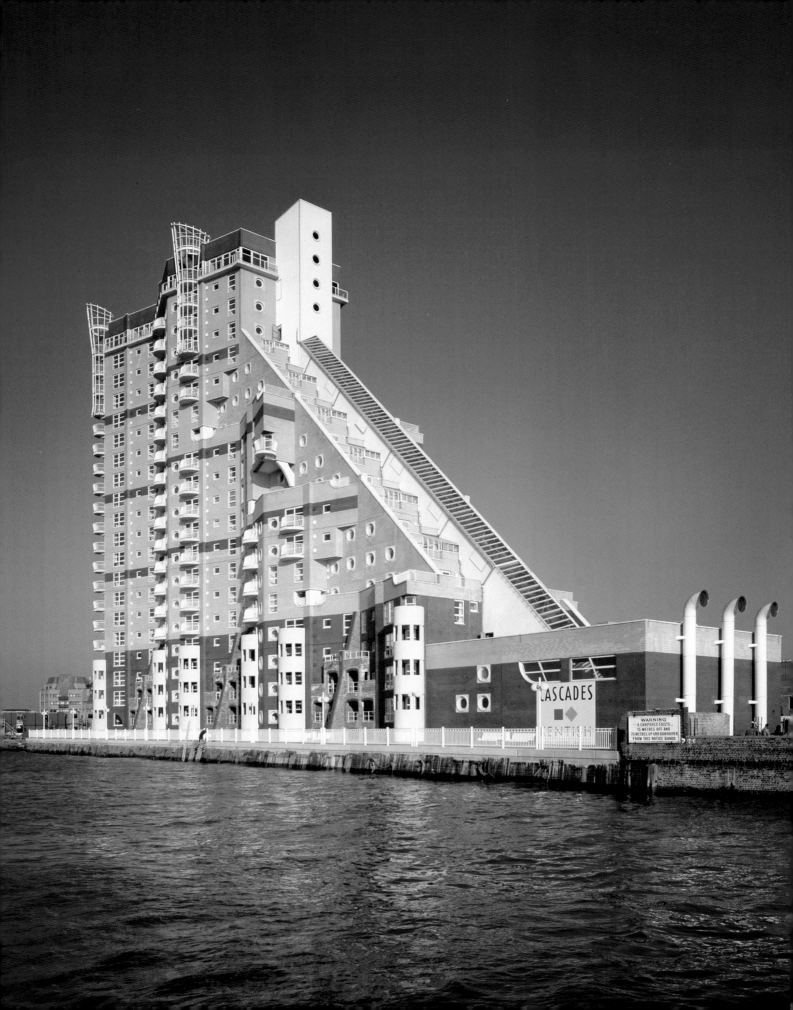

A24 CZWG, Cascades, 2-4 Westferry Road, Isle of Dogs E14, 1986-88. Built in record time, this bold ship factory-tower block was the Docklands' first high-rise housing; it has 20 storeys to the ground on the south side, and to the north, a diagonal stepped cascade of penthouses. The yellow background is broken by big bands of blue engineering brick and white features which evoke ships' bridges, portholes, turrets or an industrial escape chute. Many apartments have a superb view from their own terrace behind a little rounded balcony. Now that Canary Wharf has risen 50 storeys behind it – sober, Post-Modern Classicist and dull – this exuberant gesture makes much more sense.

A25 CZWG, The Circle, Queen Elizabeth Street SE1, 1987-90. A mixed residential/commercial development (with over 300 apartments) on two sides of a street near Butlers Wharf is finished in deep purple and blue glazed bricks. These turn the circular courtyard into a darkly shimmering, open-cast lapis lazuli mine. Quirky balconies are set on the diagonal creating a spiral motion which is echoed in the wavy roofline. The blue skin slicing across the side streets' dull yellow stock brick also makes the development a conceptual geode. And then there are the 'owl profiles' which Gough calls 'vases'. All in all the strangest mixed metaphor in London.

A26 JOHN OUTRAM ASSOCIATES, McKay Trading Estate No 1, Blackthorne Road, Poyle, Bucks, 1977-78. These warehouses show Outram's combination of Corbusian and Classical grammar and his interest in representing the translation of nature into culture, a preoccupation of many Renaissance architects including Serlio. The heavy, flat Outram arch, the polychromatic banded brick, the Classical asymmetrical symmetries are all present in this early work.

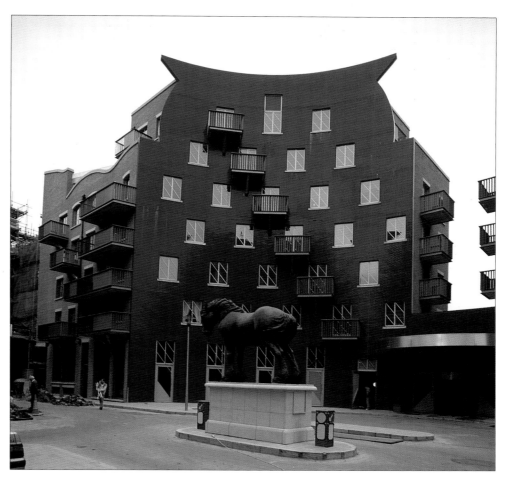

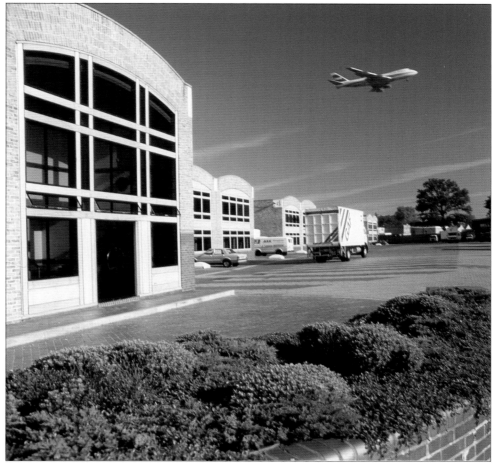

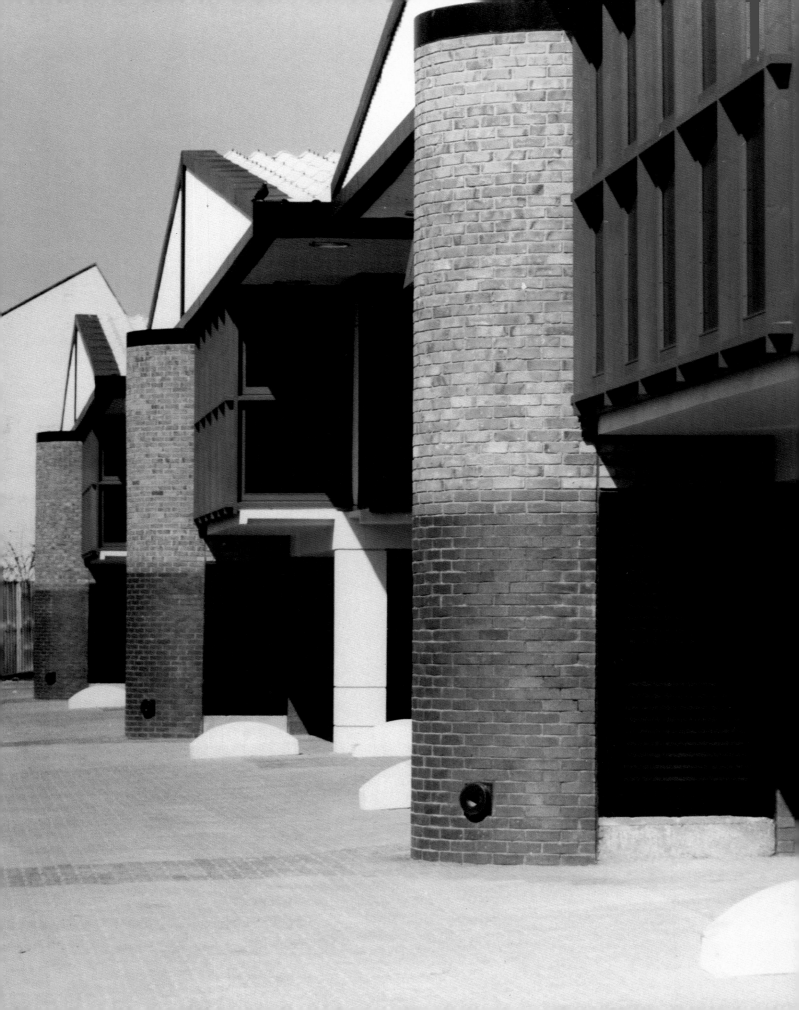

A27 JOHN OUTRAM ASSOCIATES, McKay Trading Estate No 2, Kensal Road W10, 1978-80. A Classical white pediment of corrugated metal is stretched way beyond the normal span to give what Outram calls an 'avian' image, a flying quality intensified by the hovering steel offices and main central support. Usually such utilitarian sheds are given a dumb neutrality but here, there is an ironic appropriation of a 'monostyle Order' banded rustication, an 'aedicule' or little temple and other mythic elements to root the transient functions of contemporary life (one of the sheds contains a video company).

A28 JOHN OUTRAM ASSOCIATES, Storm Water Pumping Station, Stewart Street, Isle of Dogs, 1986-88. Primitive Classicism contrasts with playful polychromy. The heaviest engaged columns in the Western world carry the most outrageous (but sensible) concrete capitals in red, yellow and blue. A revolving jet-engine of a fan breaks the bottom chord of the pediment, recalling the splits of Baroque grammar but – more to the point – giving the building its functional legibility. Outram, more than other Post-Modernists, seeks an archetypal symbolism in Modern requirements such as pumping, venting or holding the structure. It takes time before the extreme contrasts of Primitivism versus pretty ornament sink in and the viewer understands this is a new kind of grammar and meaning, intended to symbolise a river, and a landscape from which the storm-water flowed. Blue bricks signify the river, the big round red central columns represent tree trunks.

A29 JOHN OUTRAM ASSOCIATES, Blackfriar's Lane Office Infill, 200 Queen Victoria Street, Blackfriars EC4, 1991. Classical tripartition mixed with the representation of contemporary realism – in this case the railroad trains which swoosh through the middle of the building. The base has a tripartite division which culminates on the 'wheels capitals', Pop Art blue versions of Ionic volutes given a rubber-tyre bulbosity, and the green 'attic storey' turns the four superimposed 'train cars' into something more nature-like, with curves, fillets and trellis. Hence another sequential transformation, but this one from industry into culture into nature!

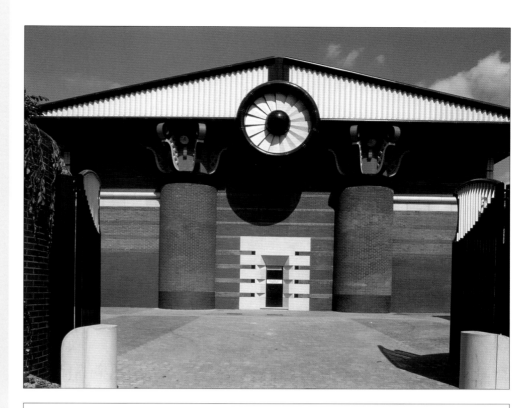

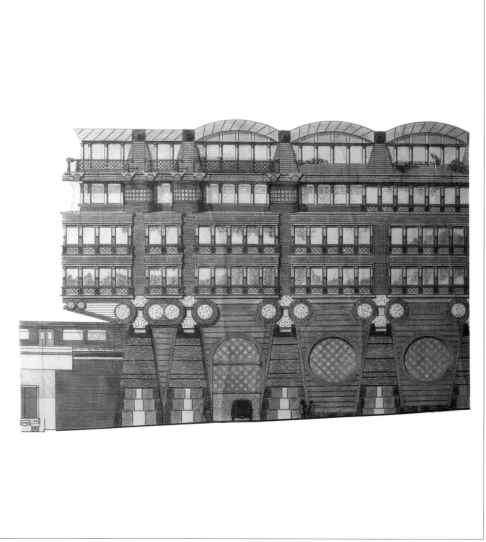

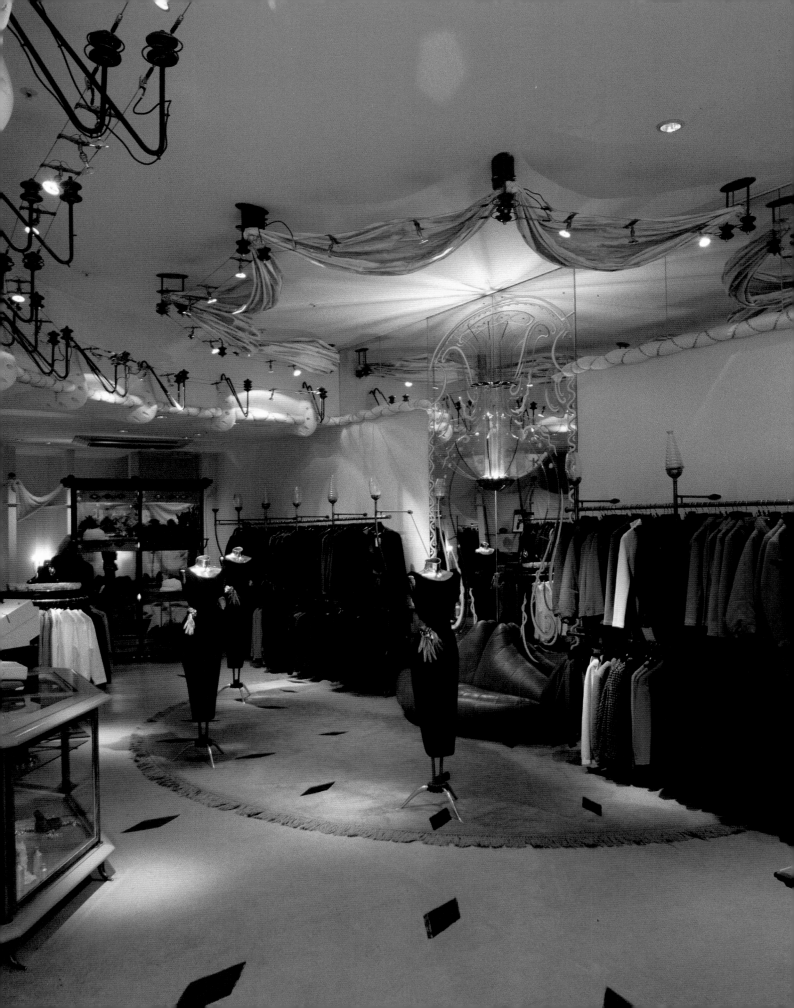

A30 BRANSON COATES ARCHITECTURE,
Katherine Hamnett Shop, 20 Sloane Street
SW1, 1988. As the architects write – 'mir-
rors, chandeliers and moulded ceilings are
distorted by exuberant misquotation: the
standard forms have been enlarged, three
dimensionalised, obscured or remade with
the painter's brush.' What they call 'an
exploded Adam ceiling' is one of these standard
forms – white fish look as if they were sliding
off the fuselage of a plaster 747. Mae West's
lips gratis *Salvador Dali* are recognisable, as
is the jumped-up Venetian mirror. Insectile
High-Tech confronts swags of decorators'
fabric, two green aquaria bookend this tiny
space. This is delirious, knowing consumer-
ism turned into a light ironic comment on
itself, the art of the non-sequitur and clothes
as instant personality.

A31 BRANSON COATES ARCHITECTURE,
Jigsaw Shop, Barkers, 65 Kensington High
Street W8, 1988. This yellow and blue ambi-
ence mixes the tough and sensual in about
equal measure. One is tempted to call it
Baroque Minimalism, or reach for any ex-
tremes to grasp the exaggerated oppositions.
The walls are of strong blue wood which has
been stripped and distressed – like an
anchorite. Shoppers trying on clothes cross
austere deserts of bare floor pulled by the
brilliant yellow sunburst at the end of the
shop (by Tom Dixon) or else aim at the Olde
English oak wardrobe. This has its doors
thrown open in abandon, as if the inhabitant
had just fled The Last Days of Brideshead. *But*
the sagging sofa cuts the mood from country
house and desert to plunge us suddenly into
the swinging 50s with flying boomerang
shapes. Then, returning to the Mediterranean theme, we find the scrolled finials
(shepherds' crooks?) and overhead the
sparkling stars (of Bethlehem?). My decoding
is too literal and aberrant, but such incon-
gruous thoughts are a direct response to
Nigel Coates' 'narrative architecture', always
a collage of technological realism, historicism,
Arts and Crafts detailing and zappy (if elusive)
imagery. If the 1980s was for some the era of
the boutique, restaurant, and simulacra then
in Coates it has found its Bernini.

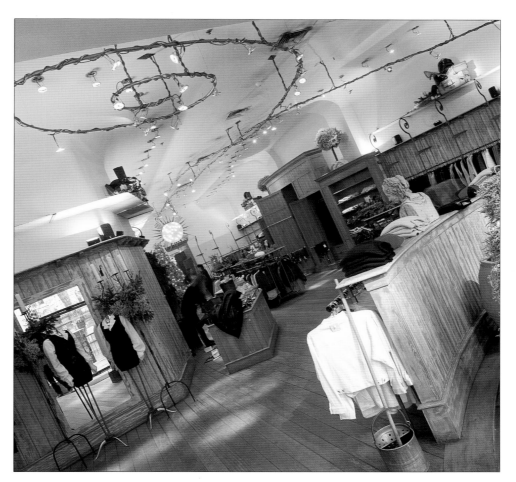

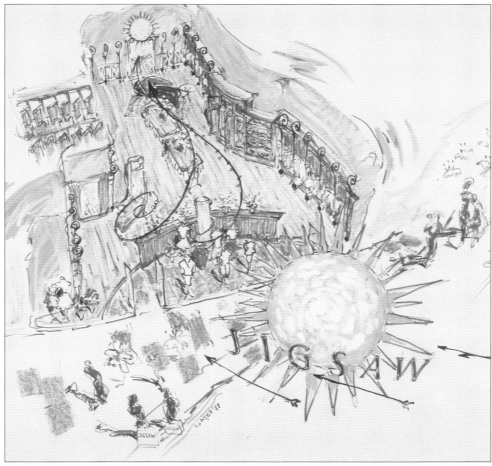

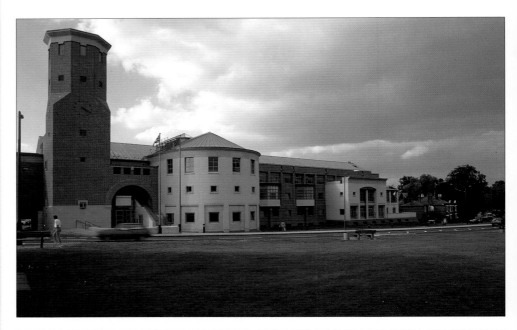

A32 *RICHARD REID, Epping Civic Centre, Epping High Street, Essex, 1982-90. A superb example of Post-Modern contextualism which pulls together a messy high street with a set of strong forms and contrasting colours (including canary yellow) that will take a little time to settle down. Give it ten years, some planting and this urban setpiece will be visually drinkable. The long, low three-storey block, contextual to the existing street scale, is anchored by a strong octagonal tower that also marks a huge arch and the main entry.*

This combination recalls Queen Anne Revival precedents but with small Rossian windows and a Gravesian flare at the top – a stone parapet. The Council Chamber curves out to the street, as it should, to call attention to the main organ of democracy and, like the Members Room, is faced in sandy reconstituted stone. The background offices are, appropriately, the same light brick as the tower. An internal courtyard in banded stone, pink and beige, and the interior of the Council Chamber complete the 'public' nature of the res publica in a sober Free-Style Classicism. Small block planning and sensible articulations also make this a minor milestone in the Post-Modern search for a legible, symbolic architecture.

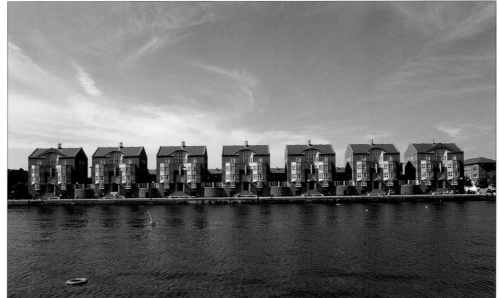

A33 *RICHARD REID ARCHITECTS, Finland Quay West, Omega Gate, off Redriff Road, Rotherhithe SE16, 1988. As in MacCormack's Shadwell Basin (A35), complex intersecting rhythms syncopate their way round a central water piazza. A long terrace of flats and maisonettes which look like houses contrasts straight London stock brick vernacular with Baroque bow fronts and large curved pediments.*

A34 *MICHAEL HOPKINS, Bracken House, 10 Cannon Street EC3, 1988-91. A sympathetic reinterpretation of Albert Richardson's reinterpretation of Guarino Guarini's reinterpretation of a Baroque Roman palazzo – the building is not the 'infinite regress' this sounds, but a highly integral completion of a game started long ago. Richardson designed the pink* Financial Times *building in 1955 in an industrial Classical Baroque manner incorporating the slight curves of the 18th-century Palazzo Carignano by Guarini. Heavy, blocky, chunky it was, but a massiveness broken by champhered corners and an even bay rhythm.*

Hopkins takes up the curves in a giant central atrium, and then swells them outwards as Guarini did – but mixing the grammar of cast iron, glass wall and bronze, the materials Richardson used. An interesting bay rhythm is created which only has the fault – of Richardson's – in being repeated a bit too remorselessly. The cornice line, heights and basic tripartition of the older decorations

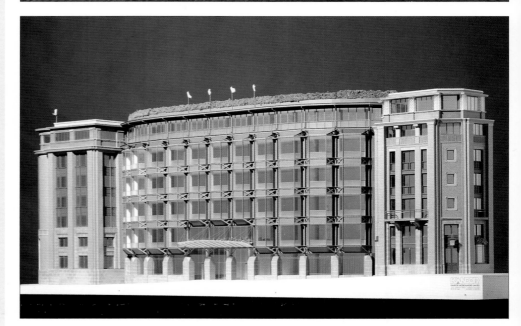

are kept, but transformed. The 'Order' of cast iron and bronze shows a previous high-tech architect moving into the Post-Modern Classical realm; Hopkins' background (coming from Foster's office) explains the repetitive sobriety of the solution: spartan, no-nonsense, almost heroic (but in the end understated).

A35 *MACCORMAC JAMIESON PRITCHARD & WRIGHT, Shadwell Basin Housing, Wapping E1, 1986-88. 169 Houses and flats massed around three sides of the old basin, once principal entrance to London Docks. This is 'Wharfism' incarnate, the recollection of the grand 19th-century tradition of industrial buildings in the Docks. Arches, porthole windows, pyramidal forms, colonnades and red and blue steel syncopate their way around a huge public realm made of water, a maritime square, a blue piazza. The brick and metal structures also reflect the interior use and the distinctions of small and large space.*

A36 *MACCORMAC JAMIESON PRITCHARD & WRIGHT, Student Residences, East Site, Queen Mary & Westfield College, University of London, Mile End Road E1, 1988-89. Typical Post-Modern Industrial Classicism using the ubiquitous V-form windows, split pediments (in corrugated metal) and opposition between brick and steel, solid and void. The adjacent Grand Union Canal is one pretext for the 'Wharfist' vernacular, here again carried out with a syncopated rhythm of reds and blues – set in a typology of six three-storey 'houses'.*

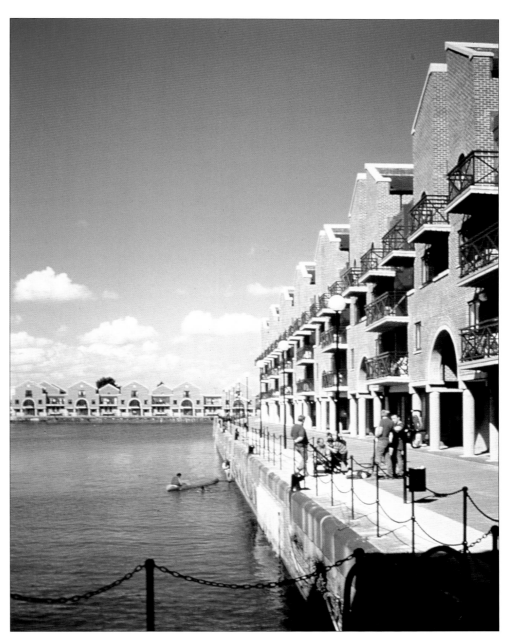

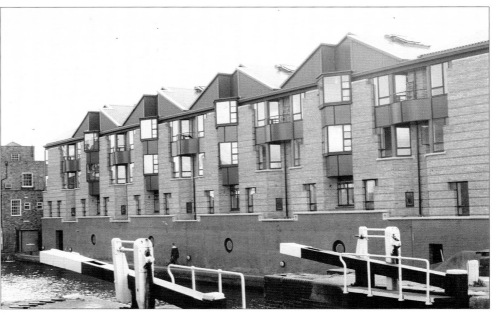

A37 MACCORMAC JAMIESON PRITCHARD & WRIGHT, Informatics Teaching Laboratory, Queen Mary & Westfield College, University of London, Mile End Road E1, 1988-89. MacCormac has done a masterful study of Frank Lloyd Wright's early grammar and it is apparent here in the details, massing and abstract symmetries. The extreme economy of the building is evident in the tight plan and the concrete is reminiscent of Wright's economies at the Unity Temple – note the corner windows, the overhanging eaves, the Rietveld-like juxtapositions of glass, metal and roof. The social cohesion of the departments is reinforced by the visual contact through the double height spaces which connect the various floors. A gem of a modest building.

A38 MACCORMAC JAMIESON PRITCHARD & WRIGHT, Housing, Vining Street, Brixton SW9, 1988-90. This residential project for the Metropolitan Housing Trust provides 75 flats, specifically designed for young, single people in an 'Inner City' environment. The scheme re-establishes previous building lines and street frontages. Problems of shared access are addressed by designing stairs as a visible part of the street scene. As in other schemes the architects are reinterpreting the single-family house typology as a suitable street form – carried out in a mixed Post-Modern Classical/Industrial style.

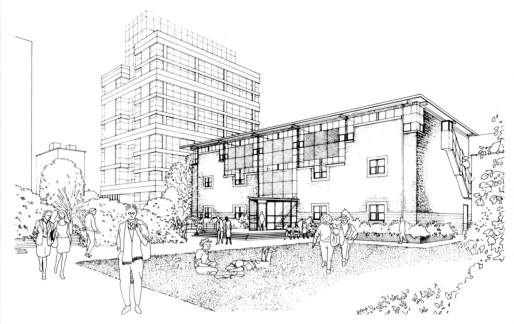

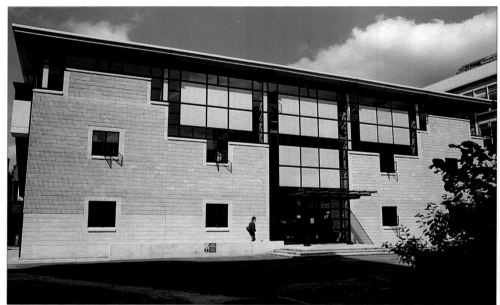

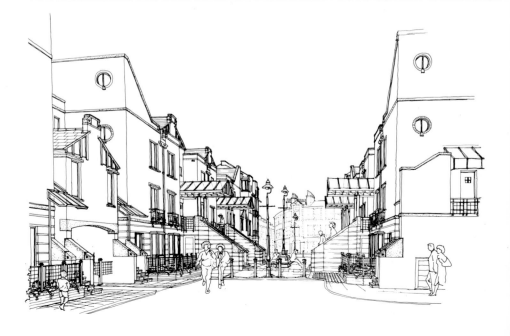

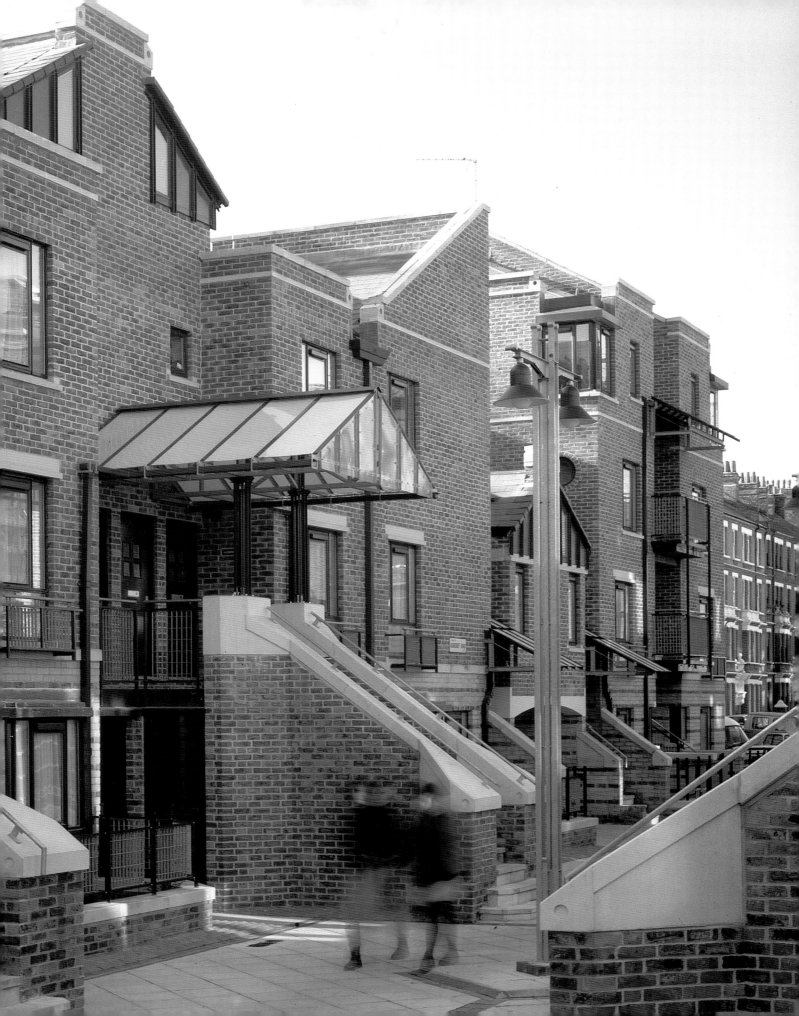

A39 *JULYAN, WICKHAM ASSOCIATES, Horsleydown Square, 1987-91. This very pleasant urban square is contained by a mixed grammar of grey concrete, yellow London stock brick, red stucco and blue steel. Above, red cylinders punctuate the skyline recalling both Italian Renaissance and Russian Constructivist forms. That double-coding is dynamic and effective, whereas the ultra-thin engaged concrete 'Order' is neither quite up to Modern nor Traditional precedents. Nonetheless the space, movement and contrasts are well paced and ultimately convincing.*

A40 *SOM, Broadgate Development, 155 Bishopsgate, EC2, 1987-91. Post-Modern Classicism combined with a Chicago industrial look. Green-tinted glass and green steel contrast sharply with the pink flesh tones and grey granite of the main body. Corner turrets act as hinges to pull commuters into Liverpool Street Station. Three huge windows with Jencksiana – head, torso, legs – divide up this massive 12-storey facade and take one's mind off its pragmatic density.*

Broadwalk House, in ruddy pink schockbeton, *resembles a soft terracotta and the even softer flesh tones of the body. Once again Chicago windows and corner 'hinges' recall the rigours of industrial Classicism in the American Midwest – the very image of what was often condemned as 'the commercial style' in 1910.*

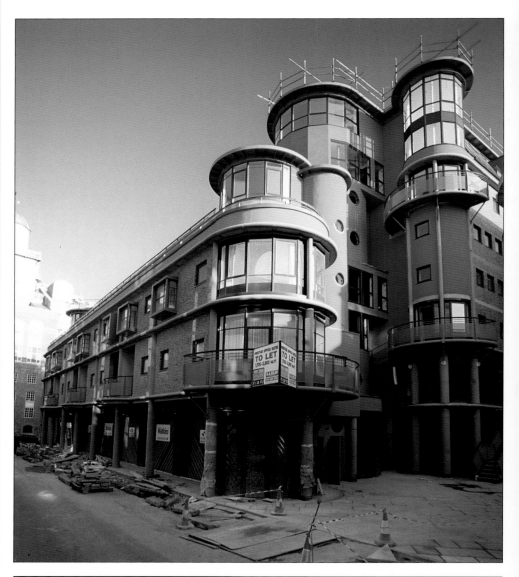

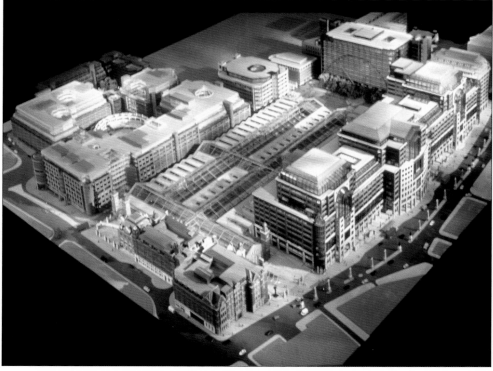

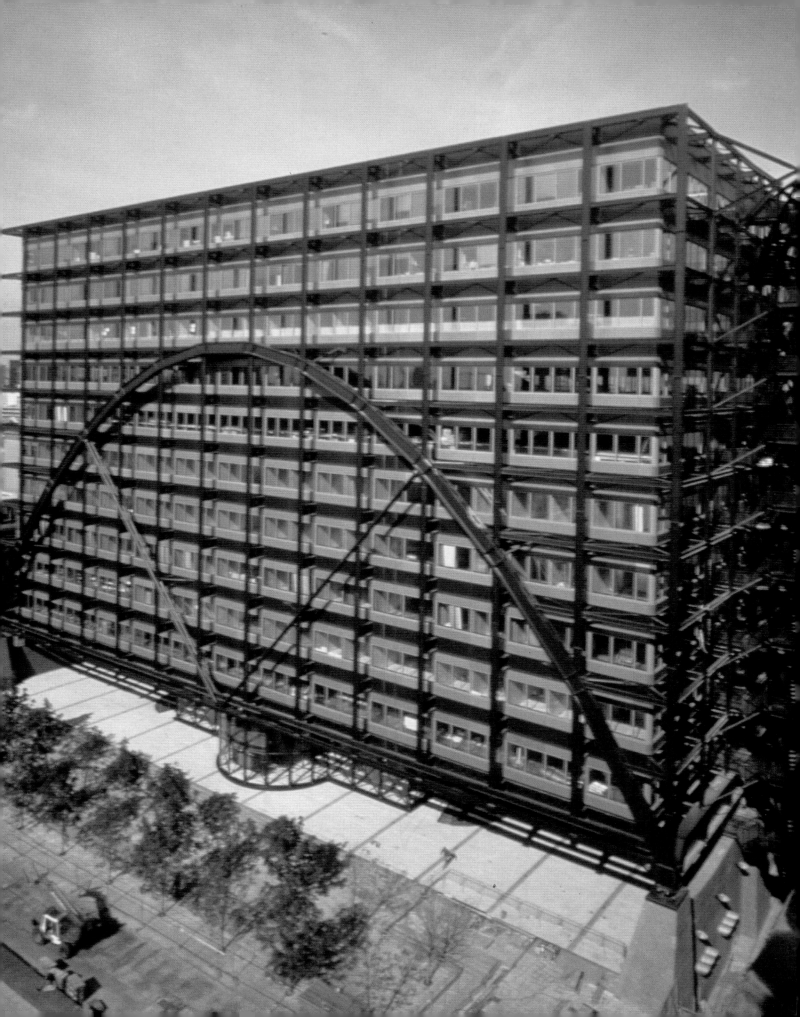

A41 SOM, Masterplanners. IM PEI; TROUGHTON McASLAN; KOHN PEDERSEN FOX; CESAR PELLI & ASSOCIATES; ALLIES AND MORRISON, Canary Wharf, Marsh Wall E14. As the panoramic view reveals, Phase One of this mega-project, due to finish in 1992, is bounded by CZWG's Cascades (far left) and Richard Rogers' Reuters (far right). Four more phases are planned if this, the biggest development in Europe, can get its transport working and the market climbs back. Otherwise it is destined to remain a suburban offshoot of the City, not its other centre and rival. Except for the tower, the architecture is mostly heavy Edwardian Classicism planned around huge Beaux-Arts circuses and squares; the kind of municipal buildings one finds in Washington DC, parts of Chicago and New York. This 'American' urbanism has been vigorously attacked by British planners, architects and critics, but in the end the doubters may come around to admiring the landscaping and urbane space. Nearest to completion are the Kohn Pedersen Fox semicircles (bottom left of the tower), marble-clad blocks with a Classical tripartition, the surface enhanced by a metal and glass screen that wraps around the middle of the south facade and through the masonry pilasters to the north. These masses have been split apart by the light railroad.

In the foreground of the perspective are SOM's curved Classical blocks surrounding Westferry Circus and fronting the Thames. This is urban wallpaper applied to big 10-storey slabs, but the open spaces, 32 species of trees, walks, terraces, water courts and endless 'street furniture' overseen by Sir Roy Strong will make it a unique place in London.

40,000 people are expected to work here in 26 different buildings, most of which are adjacent to water. A 400-bed hotel and series of mixed uses are planned: conference centre, health club, banks, post offices and medical facilities, etc. Basically Phase One is the size of Broadgate, but built at a stroke – a multi-billion pound City on the Edge of the City. Its fortunes will hang in the balance for several years. Olympia & York, big Canadian developers, have gambled and won many times, as at New York's Battery Park City – but this one is the biggest bet yet, placed anywhere. Perhaps that's why the architecture plays it so safe, more Prince Charlesesque than Post-Modernism.

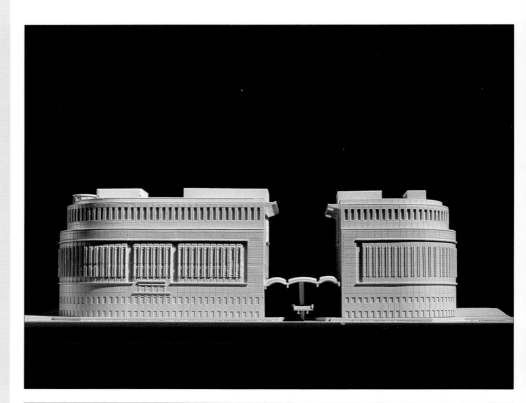

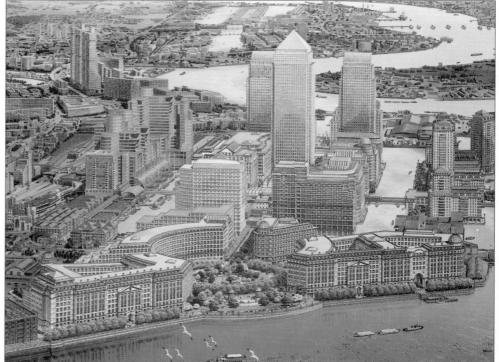

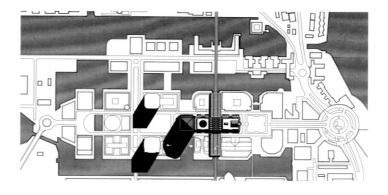

A42 *KOHN PEDERSEN FOX, Goldman Sachs Co, Peterborough Court, off Fleet Street EC3, 1988-91. This ground-scraper nestles behind* The Daily Telegraph *Building and relates its different walls and windows to the different contexts which crowd in on all sides. A heroic attempt at contextualism against all the odds – given its massive proportions – it modulates the roofline with a vaulted metal roof and pavilion. The general Post-Modern Classicism includes the usual corpus – square Rossian windows, gentle Gravesian arches, asymmetrical symmetry and lots of grey and black granite. The architects write:*

> *The formal composition of Peterborough Court implies a summary of the project's architectural context. Each of its constituent volumes assumes the scale of the structures surrounding it, combined in a way which acknowledges the picturesque, collagistic nature of the City. The two grids imposed by the site's cardinal axes and the Fleet Street structures give order to the project's asymmetry: public functions are housed in those volumes relating to Fleet Street, with the typical offices located in the body of the building, oriented on the site boundary-imposed grid. Perceptually, Peterborough Court will act as a series of discrete formal events comprehensible primarily at pedestrian scale. Its extremely impacted site and lack of frontage on Fleet Street deprive the project of any significant middle ground presence in the City. For that reason, its asymmetrical volumes have been considered as individual compositions, each responding to its immediate context. This 'pictorial' approach provides a variety of experiences for the building's users.*

> *On Fleet Street, the project is entered through the arched storefront of Mersey House, a small structure immediately east of* The Daily Telegraph *Building. Mersey House's black granite vestibule gives way to a five-storey glass gallery which runs around Peterborough Court itself, connecting the project's eastern and western entries as well. Beyond the gallery, the project's cylindrical main lobby provides access to the upper-level elevator lobby.*

A43 *CESAR PELLI & ASSOCIATES, Canary Wharf Tower, Canary Wharf, Isle of Dogs E14, 1988-91. An 800-foot, steel-clad, 50-storey tower is capped by an illuminated steel pyramid. This obelisk-like shape, Europe's tallest building for the moment, is divided up into well-proportioned sections and given a sober, repetitive surface befitting its status as 'London's Eiffel Tower'.*

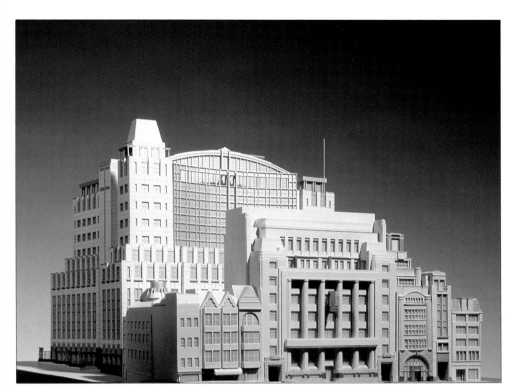

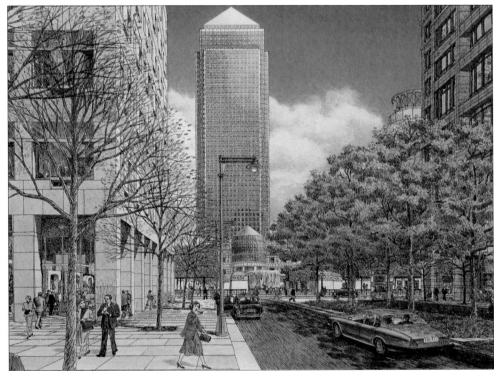

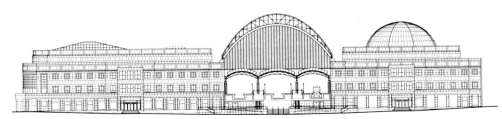

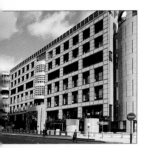

Arup's 8-12 Broadgate, 390,000 sq ft of Big Bang space is clothed on the outside with a constructed Order hung between two corner towers.

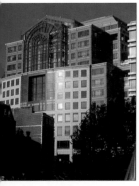

SOM's Bishopsgate Exchange, 400,000 sq ft of office is broken up by the red and white granite and green steel and glass layering.

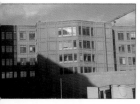

SOM's Broadwalk House, with its edible pink schockbeton, *is the contemporary equivalent of the terracotta buildings of the 1900s.*

The Broadgate development in the City of London (A40), like a slow multi-stage rocket, is reaching the end of its six-year ascent. Not a year passes without the Prime Minister launching one of its 14 stages or Torvill and Dean giving a boost to its open-air ice rink. To some, Broadgate, the largest redevelopment in the City since the Great Fire of 1666, is too broad: a monotonous repetition of red granite grilles and too much office space. But it's also an area where by late 1991, 25,000 people will commute, work, shop and play – a dense city in the City.

Prince Charles, pressed for an opinion as he launched the main square two years ago, was uncharacteristically at a loss for words and answered, 'No comment'. Some architects, annoyed by the American design of phases six to 14, have sneered 'pastiche' at the Post-Modern Classicism along Bishopsgate Road.

These reactions seem inadequate to a development which is so varied, huge and of such a grand vision that it confounds one-liners. It has been seen as a British version of Rockefeller Center because of its skating rink, pubs, restaurants and shopping arcades; or as five horizontal Empire State Buildings because of its equivalent office space; or as a set of massive 'groundscrapers', large building blocks with deep planes and central atria which reflect the new trading requirements; or as a Disneyland because the whole site is controlled, cleaned and vandal-proofed by a full-time bodyguard of 50 managers. For most people, it is simply the first conspicuous symbol of the Big Bang and the 24-hour trading world, the development that beat its dozen competitors in a race to attract the most prestigious tenants. When the sun comes out, bands play and thousands sit in the two adjoining squares, one can imagine visions of the Piazza San Marco in the architects' collective mind.

Yet these images capture only a part of the scheme which, like any decent city, is a mixture of uses, styles and ages of building. Phases one through to four, now complete, were designed by Peter Foggo of Arup Associates in a picturesque manner mixing high-tech tops with a trellis of red granite squares on the first five storeys. Although a bit remorseless – endless ice-cube grids hanging off all sides – they do break up the heavy scale into humanely-sized chunks, and they have interesting refinements. These are particularly visible on the south face of phase three, occupied by the Union Bank of Switzerland. Here is a decorative order that can stand comparison with the Gothic and Classical spec offices of the 19th century so much beloved of English Heritage and SAVE. Different sized black voids give a varied rhythm to sets of floors, and pieces of stone alternate with the clips that hold them in place to create a Post-Modern ornamental system that stems from the construction. The most stunning effect comes from the way the granite is treated – 'flame finished' on its side edges and polished on its front to a hot-dog red. As Salvador Dali claimed, all good architecture should be edible; when the sun is out here one begins to salivate.

The American-designed phases continue this sensuous quality round to the Bishopsgate side, a street which was to be lined by new lighting standards of sculpted bishops' heads. This, and the vaguely Classical ordering of arches, are the kind of details which have annoyed British Modernists who see their country succumbing to brash Chicago taste. And its 12-storey bulk does seem oppressive at first. But the architects, Skidmore Owings & Merrill, have broken up this hulk into three pavilions and given each one a large expanse of glass which conveys the implicit figure of the human body. The mixture of materials – red and white granite, green aluminium and green glass – also breaks down the scale effectively.

As one traverses this miniature city, more and more styles and building types are discovered. There is the heart of the scheme, the old Liverpool Street train sheds of 1875, now repainted and brought back to their Neo-Gothic, polychromatic splendour. No doubt their mixture of 19th-century high-tech and religious fretwork have inspired Skidmore Owings & Merrill on the Bishopsgate side of their buildings. But where these offices sit over the tracks, or confront the station directly, they change style again and become, like the trains and sheds, abstract and industrial. Phase 11, now virtually complete, rises from four gigantic parabolic arches, the most notable example of structural expressionism in London until Norman Foster gets to work (for the same developers) at Kings Cross.

There are several more styles, and phases, near completion and the most accomplished in traditional terms is hidden away in the north corner of the site. Broadwalk House, as it is known, again has an overall reddish hue, but it is made from a special concrete called *schockbeton* which is so finely grained, warm and homogeneous that it feels, on touch, like the built equivalent of skin. For this giant 'hinge' building the architects have adapted the Chicago office style and a very delicate ornamental pattern that is reminiscent of turn-of-the-century buildings in that city.

With 14 buildings, a variety of styles, uses and public squares, Broadgate has an urbanity missing from other recent mega-buildings. This is the lasting contribution of the scheme. One only has to think of the monotonous slabs at London Wall or the depressing homogeneity of the Barbican to see how far we have come in 25 years. From anonymous curtain walls to ornamented clip-on facades, from streets in the air to pedestrian alleyways on the ground, from single use to multiple functions – these are the values for which Post-Modernists have fought. Only the desire for small scale is disappointed. And the large size, ultimately two billion pounds worth of building, is the price we have to pay for the public amenities and urban space. As the developer Stuart Lipton says, the public realm has to be *funded*, either by the State or the client – and today one knows which that will be.

In the 60s era of such developments as Harry Hyams' Centre Point, there was little regard for aesthetics or urban amenities. Speed of building and profit were the motives. Today developers are aware, as Lipton puts it, that 'good architecture sells and rent-slabs don't'. Broadgate was the result of intensive market research over several years which revealed the demand for high quality office space. This demand was so great in London in the late 1980s that it led to a dozen or so comparable schemes under construction and an increase of one-third in City office space. Much of this was expected to rent at high prices – 40 pounds per square foot – in spite of the Big Bang collapse and the slide in the stock market. Since the major banks, such as Chase Manhattan, have laid off hundreds of traders, the building boom has spluttered along through the market bust – at least when the new office space offers enough quality.

Lipton compares Broadgate to a BMW and the prestigious tenants it attracts to a fashion-conscious woman who wants something sexy – a health club, a lively place to meet people, a park. Hence the many amenities and continuous events in the public square, the commissioned sculpture of Segal, Serra and Bottera, and the polished granite benches placed in a square of cobblestones and plane trees. The formula is meant to cure 'yuppie burnout', or too many hours at the video screen watching the Tokyo and New York markets bounce up and down. It's only fitting that, to attract and keep City workers, Mammon now has to provide public space, site-specific sculpture, wine bars, continuous sideshows of concerts and skating, and acceptable urbanism. That's Post-Modern progress over the Modern city, even if it's not quite the Piazza San Marco.

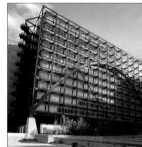

Broadgate, aerial axonometric, shows the 13 phases of building surrounding Liverpool Street Station to the south and thus becoming a metaphorical 'broadgate' to this city entrance. Urbane values are apparent – the way public squares, alleys and streets are threaded through the scheme and the variety of styles. Also visible is the Big Bang deep floor plan with its central atrium and skylight – a Post-Modern type of the late 80s which allowed the City to have its information revolution surrounded by greenery and plenty of light.

SOM's Phase 11, the bridge building, suspended over the way train tracks on four parabolic arches, is also suspended over an open ground floor to create an operatic entrance to a stepped water garden. The black, technocratic image is a pleasant contrast to the adjacent Free-Style Classicism and semantically appropriate to Liverpool Street Station on which it looks.

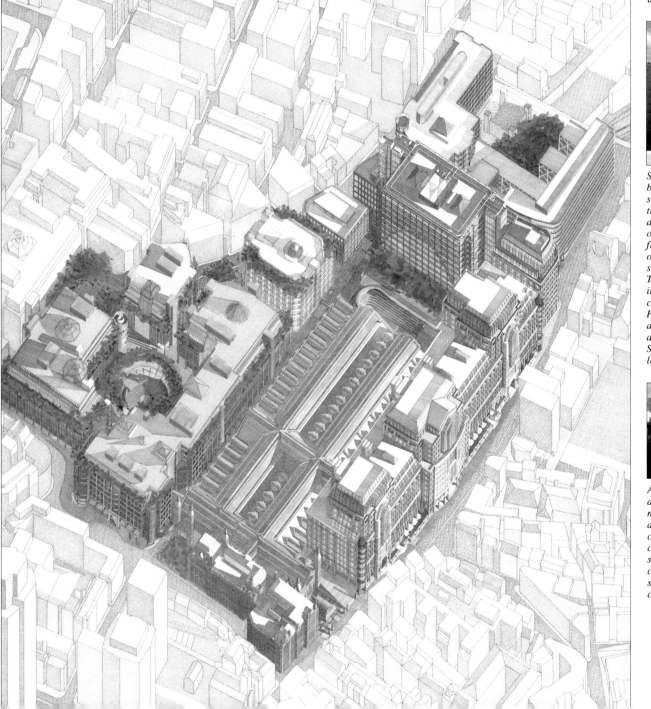

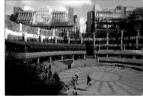

Arup's Broadgate Arena, an amphitheatre for music, spectator sports and skating, takes a circular form and colonnade and then softens these essentially classical forms with screens, planting, chamfers and asymmetry.

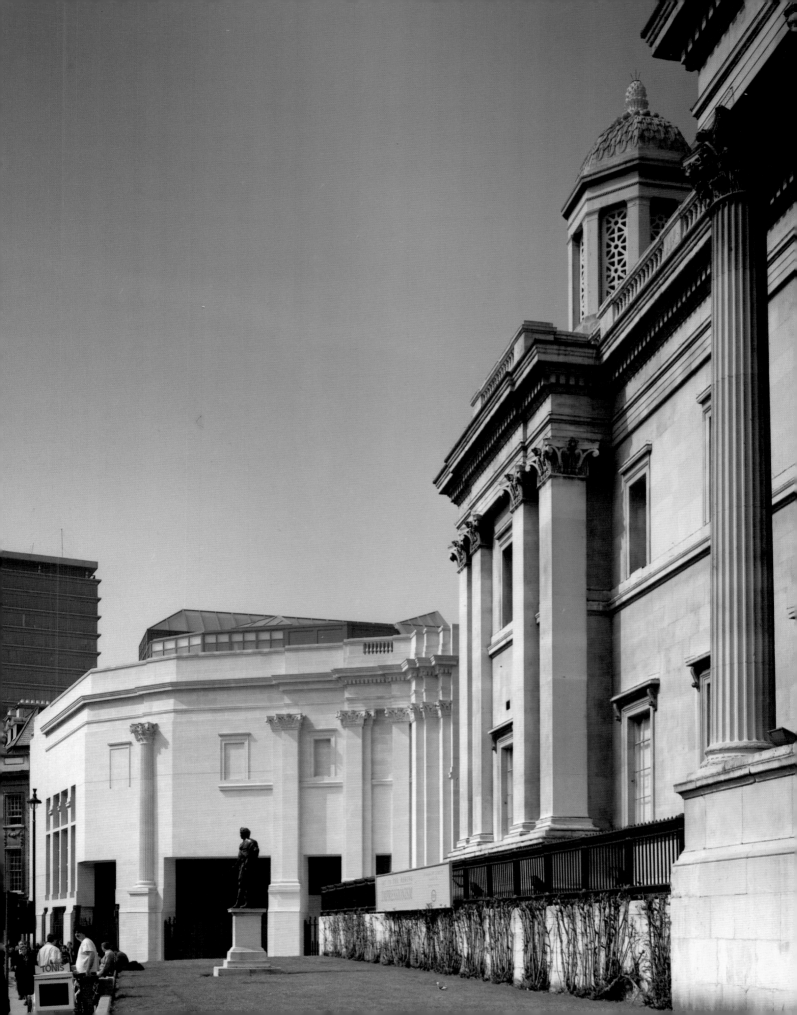

NATIONAL GALLERY – SAINSBURY WING
ROBERT VENTURI, DAVID VAUGHAN & CHARLES JENCKS
An Interview

The Museum as Popular Institution

Charles Jencks: Paul Goldberger said, when you got the commission for the National Gallery addition, that it was one of the 'most significant in Europe ever awarded to an American architect'. Of course there's IM Pei's pyramid.

Robert Venturi: I don't like to be *too* conscious of a historical position. For instance, when I wrote *Complexity and Contradiction in Architecture*, I didn't connect its content with the naming of a style – I leave that to historians or theoreticians like you. But it is an important institution in an important location in an important country. Where it will stand in history – I just forget about that . . .

CJ: I was thinking of it as a characteristic building type – that strange but significant shift in the 80s to modest additions to huge museums.

David Vaughan: Strangely, as an addition it has almost all the functions of a complete building within it – restaurant, auditorium – many of the things they never had in the original building, and now want.

RV: A lot of the functioning spaces of the original building are on the ground floor – which the public never goes to – but the loading and service areas of our addition have to be sized to serve the entire National Gallery. Our wing is like an organism separate from the older building, which has glandular problems where some of its elements must serve the whole complex.

When you're planning museums – and we have been designing them in Seattle, San Diego and Texas – you find that only one-third of the space is dedicated to exhibitions. The rest is given over to didactic use and administration requirements.

CJ: It's also because vast numbers of people come through the National Gallery – three million – and they want an art education.

RV: Yes, it's the result of galleries today being popular places.

DV: It's also the only place The National Gallery can expand: they even wanted to put more functions on that site, but it wasn't possible.

A Walk around the 'Five' Facades: the First Facade

CJ: I'd like to take you around what I'd call the 'five' facades, starting with the main entrance. The most striking aspect of the Sainsbury Wing, which you feature in perspectives, is the oblique approach from Trafalgar Square – the continuation of the Corinthian Order in staccato syncopation at the corner so that it culminates in a pulsating line of about 20 of Wilkins' columns and pilasters. Why this

figure on the 'first' facade?

RV: We enjoyed being contextual – to use an over-used word. As a small building facing a big space it has to make some kind of gesture toward Trafalgar Square – to fill up that corner and reinforce enclosure. It has to read as part of the old building but separate from it too. As it evolves toward the left, to what you might call the 'second' facade, it becomes part of Pall Mall and there you have another kind of scale and imagery, that of the Clubs. As to the main entrance facade, the question was at first to achieve unity either by being analogous, or by being contrasting, to the setting: we chose the more difficult role of making the addition essentially analogous to the old building, but with parts within the overall being very contrasting. At the Oberlin Museum addition we played the easier game of virtually total contrast. And here we couldn't be, as St Martin in the Fields is toward the east, a unified whole.

Also when you see The National Gallery obliquely, rather than straight-on, it *does* have enough pilasters – it's dynamic. So we decided to make the oblique view of the old building the equivalent of a straight-on elevation of the new.

The porch of the old building was for a few 'élitists', the 500 persons per day who went up the steps originally. Our building – not quite a sports stadium – still has to acknowledge that many more people come through the entrance than in 1830. No longer just gentlemen, but thousands of students on cheap air-fares.

So a few dissonant elements –

CJ: – The cuts in the base and Classical grammar?

RV: They are very big openings that acknowledge it isn't the kind of entrance which has a small porch with a few small doors in the back.

CJ: It's a very Late-Modernist door – the pronounced absence of a wall.

RV: You're absolutely right.

CJ: I've always loved your ghost pilasters – crunched up to such optical effect at the corner. They remind me of the 'out of focus' ghost pilasters at Weingarten – which make you clean your glasses – you can't count them, like Op Art they vibrate.

RV: Yes, I like Weingarten, and its anti-Neo-Classicism in its dynamic rhythmic results. It is very Baroque to cluster the columns.

CJ: But they never clustered so many in a row.

RV: Not quite, but almost. I don't know who did that

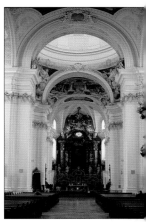

Weingarten Abbey Church, begun 1719-20 '. . . out of focus pilasters'.

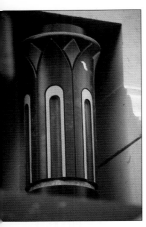

Neo-Egyptian Order?

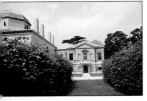

Chiswick House 'has Palladio with great chimneys popping out of the roof.'

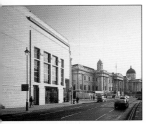

The second facade shifts in scale and order to a more sober rhythm, which relates to Canada House and the clubs.

clustering first; it might have been Michelangelo on the Campidoglio.

CJ: I think the Romans first used ghosts.

RV: Anyway, it's interesting to use that device in a very Neo-Classical context, because it isn't correct. We got that idea very quickly. Steve Izenour and I were standing in Trafalgar Square, on the second day of thinking about the project, and the contextual limitations, which are very important, guided us immediately. The idea of using the metal colonnettes, an 1830s elemental which Wilkins doesn't use, comes from the need to get small detail down at the base.

CJ: I find the Neo-Egyptian Order questionable – why didn't you create, like Adam, a new 'British Order of the National Gallery'?

RV: We didn't think much about the symbolism – we just wanted a lot of detail there at eye-level. And at that time, in the 1830s, you did combine in an arbitrary way lots of eclectic things. I don't mind being a little loose with the symbolism. After all, the whole idea of using Classicism in the English Renaissance must have been horrifying – Gibbs using a *pagan* temple as a church.

CJ: Except there was an unbroken tradition, and that's a real difference. Even before Inigo Jones there was a Bastardised Classicism – what I would call 'Mannersance'.

RV: I was reminded of the 19th-century use of the Egyptian Order while looking at Alexander 'Greek' Thomson. I adore him.

Double-Coding and Answering the Critics

CJ: That's justification enough. You went through 15 model studies to get this facade – the Modern jazz of the clustered pilasters creates a terrific tension across the opening. This is broken to reveal a black Miesian glass to one side. So you set up a series of extreme contrasts throughout the building – and play them with incredible understatement, so many people won't see them. But there's a violent Mannerist contrast – almost 'tragic *terribilità*' – as if you are saying Modernist and Traditionalist cultures are interwoven but have nothing to do with each other.

RV: In Wilkins' time there was the tradition of the conservatory, an early form of a Crystal Palace, sitting next to heavy Classical forms – so this juxtaposition connects with a tradition. Brunel's industrial bridges are suspended from massive masonry Egyptian bases.

CJ: You're giving a precedent, but my question is: Do you see this juxtaposition as a comment on the dual culture of our time?

RV: That's a good point. I think we are at a stage where eclecticism and pluralism are appropriate, but what annoys me now is the Deconstructive architecture that is *all* dissonance. When everything is dissonant, there is no dissonance. You need a norm to vary as well as a functional basis for contradiction. For instance, the black window-wall came out of the interior needs – the idea that as you go up the grand stair you borrow the Wilkins' facade for one side and create a somewhat dissonant version of

Mies van der Rohe for the other so that you connect with the red facade beyond. But it's also a simple idea – that of the building connecting with its setting and being a fragment.

CJ: What about the blackness – it reminds me of the Museum of Modern Art.

RV: It comes from tinting the glass – energy conservation – and protecting the paintings, and avoiding colour before you see the paintings.

DV: We had to bring the light level down by the stairs, as you went into the galleries, because they are going to be much darker – for conservation needs.

CJ: The problem with your double-coding is it outrages both the Modernists – who don't take your functionalism seriously and call it pastiche – and the Straight Revivalists, who find too many ironies. You've been criticised by Gavin Stamp for not playing it straight, and by Modernists for being 'capricious', 'quirky', 'contrived'. Can one ever give an answer to these kind of ideological criticisms?

RV: All I can say to the Traditionalists is 'Thank God Classicism has always been innovative and changing'. It was absurd for Gibbs to take a Roman temple and surmount it with a medieval steeple albeit in Classical garb – that was extremely shocking. It soon became the prototype for churches in America. The pilaster – the idea of using a column decoratively – must have been shocking the time it was first used. A lot of such Classical usages – which I mention in an article in the *RSA Journal* (January 1988) – must have been originally outrageous, before becoming conventional.

CJ: But the Traditionalists say the building is quirky because you take a blind window and suddenly drop the sill, or you end the Corinthian pilaster rhythm with a half engaged column which holds nothing. They're saying this is too contrived, because you should open up the blind windows – to allow light in – and end the theme not with a fade-out but a bang.

RV: I don't have a specific rebuttal for that. But the strength of Classicism is that it *does* evolve. The English especially have known this, because a good deal of their Classical history is Mannerist and quirky and at the edge of being provincial. Sometimes its Mannerism is the result of great sophistication in transforming the imported Italian architecture. It's such an irony that they should go on like this in the land that invented the fragmented ruin, 'The Romantic Ruin' (England's most original architectural contribution).

CJ: As to provincial rectitude and invention, they say 'If you want to study Rome, go to Romania'. Here they are annoyed when Americans, like you, understand English traditions better than the natives. People in a tradition need, as you say, 'creative forgetfulness' in order to get on. So they're piqued at being taught their own home truths.

I was surprised when the Georgian Group, and others who ought to know better, wanted you to lower your skylights – pull them below the brim of your cornice. That goes against so many Georgian conventions and those of Nash, where a functional, heterogeneous expression of non-architecture (chimneys, gutters and so forth) erupts above the cornice line. How could they have forgotten those special rules of misrule?

RV: Go to Chiswick and Mereworth and you have Palladio with great chimneys popping out of the roofs – the traditionalists must be humiliated, horrified. I've learned more about Classicism in England than anywhere else (after Italy), because it is the idiosyncratic, Mannerist tradition of *twisting* the Classical vocabulary that's been the most vital aspect of architecture in this country. To me the main strength is not the canons of historical architecture, but the fact the canons allow you to divert and to go off from them. That's very different from the Deconstructionists and Modernists today where *everything* is dissonant. You have to refer to a norm in the first place before you break the rules.

CJ: What is read as a weakness in the facade is the way things dissipate or fade-out but I would argue it's a very *strong* fade-out with a climax of an engaged column, and then a blend. However some Modernists are wilfully misinterpreting this through ideological glasses labelling you a 'pasticheur' – although they know perfectly well this is a very creative and appropriate solution. This is one of the most creative buildings in Britain.

The 'Second' Facade
CJ: If we continue our walk towards the left and Pall Mall – you say the facade shifts in scale, and Order to a more sober rhythm, which relates to Canada House and the Clubs. You mention a big Regency window – but I see here, again, very strong contrasts between white Portland stone and black glass.

RV: In the original design we made the window mullions whitish and later I said let's make them dark or blackish in the manner of Nash. They will probably be re-coloured so you can see their configuration and how the proportions relate directly to Wilkins' windows. We've done this like Pop Art – blowing up a convention in scale.

CJ: The black continues the strong contrast and increases the *gravitas* – if that's not too pompous a word.

RV: The Clubs also have a kind of plain-wall severity. We love the play of a facade which is twisted *à la* Aalto; indeed the character of a facetted facade (in plan) evolved from him. Also a gallery does not allow windows, the main elements in architecture that give character and show whether a building is Gothic or Renaissance or whatever. So we made up for that absence by connecting with the context.

The 'Third' and 'Fourth' Facades
CJ: You describe Whitcomb Street as 'Dickensian' and represent that in beige brick, Portland stone and metal. All of the rhythms which you see in the first two facades become so subtle – very thin slits which mark the transition between brick and stone – that they may be lost to the public (and Gavin Stamp). Some have found it, in model form, a 'boring Modernist facade'. What do you say to your critics who find it too understated and British for them to see?

RV: I would agree with them if I were they – because they are *not* yet seeing the base of the facade, including the colonnettes and capitals. If you just look at the top you will

say 'boring' – because you need the detail at eye level. They ought to withhold their criticism until they see the whole.

There is a long tradition of buildings which have 'Queen Anne Fronts and Mary Anne Behinds' as the Americans say.

CJ: But why a Mary Anne Behind on Whitcomb Street – it's more public and heavily travelled than a mews situation? Whereas the St Martin's Street facade, the rear of the museum which you've described as strong and reticent, is a real Behind situation.

RV: We'll have plane trees there which connect you to those in the courtyard – like the colonnettes, something at eye level which gives a play of detail and ornament. People should hold off criticism until the hoardings are down and they see all this detail; it's like criticising a surgeon when he's halfway through an operation and all the guts are hanging out. On the other hand, I love some of the criticism – the positive, that of JM Richards and also some negative. We've hung some above our boards: 'The facade is Picturesque, Mediocre Slime'; or, 'Again we are to receive another piece of vulgar American Post-Modern Mannerist Pastiche' – you've got to admire critics like that.

CJ: On St Martin's Street you have this big sign – 'The National Gallery' – skewered on each side by two exhaust vents; so again there are the extreme contrasts between Modernist Realism and Classical ornament. But the latter is now incredibly sweet, even pretty, almost Adamesque.

RV: A lot of this comes from particular circumstances. The panel and big letters derived from some urban design requirements of The Royal Fine Arts Commission: it's amusing that we get our own words, of many years ago, back from such bodies. There is also the element of the gates and Jubilee Walk – this whole dimension of detail which people haven't yet seen – which is extremely important.

The 'Fifth' Facade
CJ: The oval or elliptical bridge over Jubilee Walk is rather like the Bridge of Sighs in Venice.

RV: In some ways it's more a kind of connecting pavilion than bridge, set on piers, because a bridge has an arch and proclaims its spanning function. Again the tripartite window refers to the old building and again the windows should be white so that the Regency-style reference would be more explicit.

CJ: The pavilion is a 'gateway' from Leicester to Trafalgar Square?

RV: Yes, then you have the real cast iron gates at the end – which I love because of their flattened, historical configuration. They will be open during the day.

CJ: That'll be rather nice and ceremonial, to swing the gates to show the museum is open.

RV: Then of course there are a lot of gates in that big opening on Trafalgar Square, because it really makes sense in terms of the urban context.

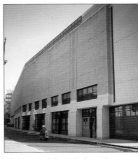

Third and fourth facades – there are very thin slits which mark the transition between brick and stone.

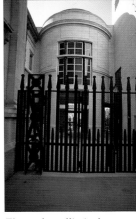

The oval or elliptical bridge over Jubilee Walk is rather like the Bridge of Sighs in Venice.

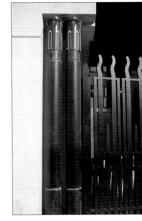

Real cast iron gates with their flattened, historical configuration.

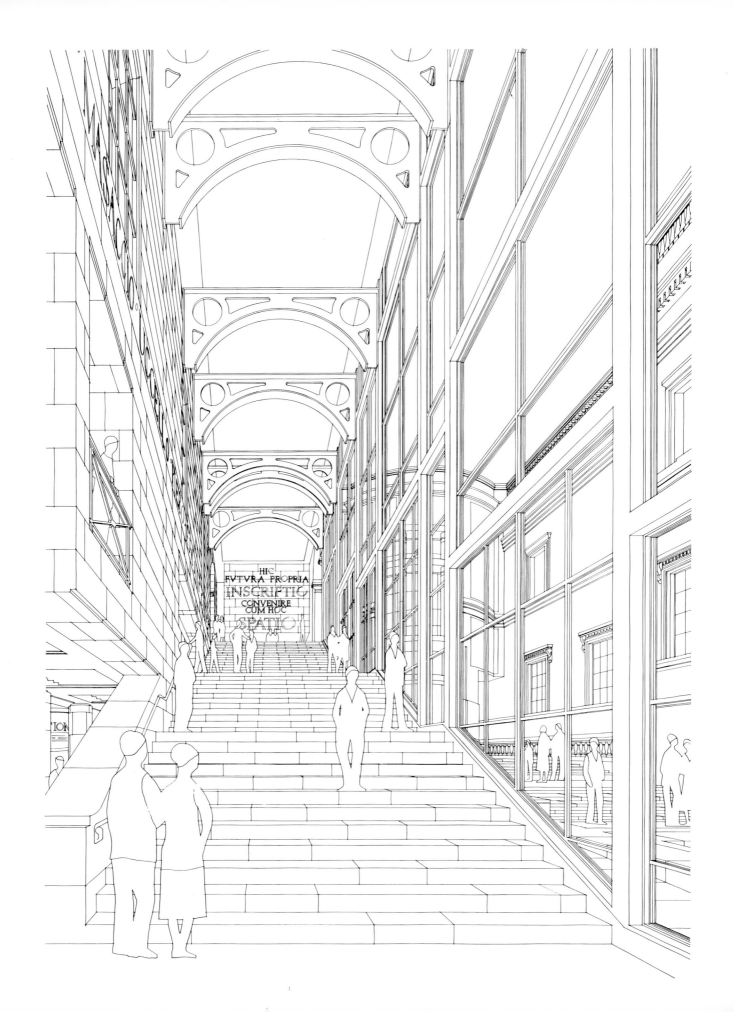

The Foyer and Processional Route

CJ: The entrance foyer has an ambiguous sliding space that gently pushes you right towards the stair – past a colonnade is it? It's a strange space which provokes Modernists because it's kind of Aalto-esque (but not quite) and provokes Classicists because it's non-figural (but almost). What does it do?

RV: There are two determinants that effect the design of this space. It is very low from necessity, because of the need to link with the elevation of the *piano nobile* of the old building; also we refer to the traditional way of dealing with a high-Classical building at ground level. In many English country houses you come into the lower part, which is designed in the manner of the outside vocabulary of the building; and then climb to the major floor above. In Italy it was often where the carriage drove in. So we gave it that character, to some extent, with the big piers.

CJ: It's a Palladian basement with sliding space. But why doesn't it form a figural void?

RV: To direct you to the elevators, to the downstairs, or up the stairs. We intend to use signs as little as possible. One of the biggest problems in a contemporary museum is that the art is remote. In the old days art greeted you at the front door, whereas now you enter into a shop and go to the lecture theatre, or administration area and so forth – you are not even sure you are in a museum. Thus you make a progression from the front door to the art and that tempts some architects to make the procession too dramatic. Actually going up the stairway is quite jazzy, but not too much. The danger of too much jazz is that, by the time you get to the art, you're worn out. It's an anti-climax, as if you've been, as I say, ejaculated through the original space.

CJ: So your foyer is a non-space after a non-door.

RV: That's right, it's a non-space and there are no doors, there's just a deep shadow at the entrance. There are a whole lot of little things to do – you can leave your coat and get information, etc – but we wanted to make a contrast as you ascend, with the traditional galleries above, those cells of enclosed space. We weren't doing a historically consistent building.

CJ: I'm very glad you explained that, because now I see it quite differently – as a transitional space. Conceptually, one always expects to go through a door and be welcomed, but you're saying the welcome is really the grand staircase and that you just get through the entrance space as quickly as possible.

RV: You are in a fragmentary directive space until you get up to the top and that makes it more wonderful up there.

The Grand Staircase

CJ: You go up the grand staircase, past the names of the Renaissance painters on the one side and black glass on the other, and you travel in reverse perspective. Here you get again the extreme contrasts between Modern and Traditional codes, High and Low Taste, modest and grand space. This is one of the most important rooms in the building (or one of the reasons you won the competition) – is it a culmination?

RV: Well naturally the most important spaces are for the paintings, and everything defers to them.

CJ: What about the Renaissance names versus the black glass – are people going to find that schizoid?

DV: You won't perceive it as black glass from the inside – because the outside will be so much brighter. And at night the black glass will disappear and all you'll see are the names and the frieze.

CJ: You'll feel between two stone walls?

RV: Yes, and you have these big English windows overlooking the stairs – like being in a cortile, both within and without.

DV: You almost go back outside after the entrance floor, because of the great amount of light.

CJ: The staircase looks to be a little bit of an anti-climax focusing on an elevator and not a work of art.

RV: But you don't see the elevator doors till you're half way up because they're recessed and not within your perspective. Functionally we had to bring everybody together at this point, a brilliant part of the plan, if I may say so – which will have big graphics and be, in effect, a billboard. Or, I wouldn't mind a very big *bas relief* there, or a big and bold enough Della Robbia.

The Post-Modern Sensibility

CJ: On the staircase you have that quintessential Post-Modern feeling of being at home in the 20th *and* the 15th century. Of course there is juxtaposition, but you feel these are equally familiar periods which are behind you, and *not* on your back. Rarely do you find architecture taking from two different epochs in a straightforward way – that Mies and Brunelleschi are both OK. Stirling at Stuttgart may play a similar game, but he dramatises the battle between taste cultures.

RV: Yes, we are in the land of eclecticism and the English who, in making one garden pavilion Greek and the next Gothic and then Indian, have consciously mixed styles since the 18th century – and to a great extent that eclectic consciousness *is* the London we see today ... It's also Tokyo today, which also interests me – another capital city with a global outlook. Our mixture involves, therefore, fitting into a tradition, and even pastiche is a word you can twist into having a good meaning – but I would use the word collage (which means in effect 'good pastiche').

CJ: If I may say, you're in danger of doing what a lawyer does – justifying by precedent – and this actually obscures the originality of your contribution and how it differs from Stourhead and l9th-century eclecticism. The distinct aspect of the Post-Modern period, and the *tension* of our time, is that we have contradictory ideas and tastes which are equally valid and not resolvable. They reflect actual social and cultural tensions – even metaphysical realities – and that was not what Stourhead and eclecticism were trying to do (which is more to put things in their place, more like a shopper).

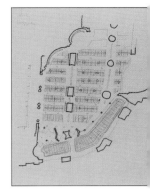
53

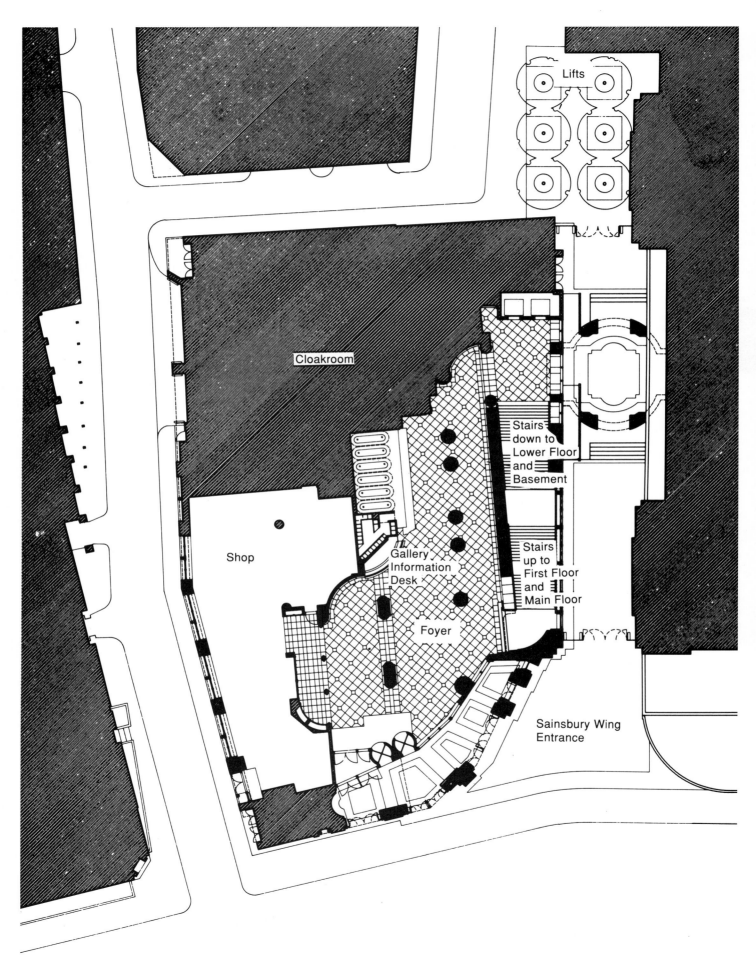

Lifts

Cloakroom

Shop

Gallery
Information
Desk

Foyer

Stairs
down to
Lower Floor
and
Basement

Stairs
up to
First Floor
and
Main Floor

Sainsbury Wing
Entrance

The Galleries

CJ: After the elevators you turn left through another false perspective, but now in the direction you're going – what does it focus on?

RV: A big Venetian altarpiece. The vestibule will have some didactic introduction, then immediately to the left is a series of 14th-century paintings, while beyond that are the central galleries with galleries of later period paintings. Those rooms have high arches which were to focus on a Palladian window with another window behind – and partial view to Pall Mall East – and to our great regret it was removed. Curators love more than anything in the world to sacrifice their great paintings for the ends of vistas.

There is a tension between the main axial views – and chronology. A new museum in Munich has quite a picturesque composition with a very specific route that is chronological; ours is more in the tradition of an old museum, where there is some chronology but also the opportunity to plan your own route.

CJ: Well, isn't it a matrix where you can have chronology going one way, and cross-cultural comparisons going the other way, a double reading? You won the competition partly because you showed interest in the art – can you say something about it?

RV: Well, I can't say much, but I'm always amused when I go into that collection. I begin laughing, because so many of the paintings are so familiar, because you've grown up seeing so many reproductions of these famous paintings. Naturally the Mannerist ones interest me a lot – and one Michelangelo I adore.

We acknowledged the client wanted something that paralleled the original setting the painters might have anticipated for their art. The sense of place was important. Also it is thrilling to see art in the real world, rather than in a museum: if you go to someone's house and they have a great painting in their living room, there is something *more* wonderful about it than if you see it in a museum – it's in the real world. At the same time you have to acknowledge the museum as an institution for accommodating high security and great crowds, so what we did was to place occasional windows in the galleries. A window indicates that you are part of the living world. Also you can look through it – and the magic you've been experiencing looking at great paintings becomes more magical after it is interrupted by the real world; it's like intermissions between acts at the theatre.

CJ: Where?

RV: There are 'Anglo-Saxon' windows to the left over the staircase as you ascend but on a huge scale.

DV: In the galleries you can go to these windows, with their window seats, and look out obliquely onto Trafalgar Square through the outer black glass.

CJ: The galleries are a silver grey?

RV: They consist of the greenish-grey Pietra Serena stone trim that Brunelleschi used in his Renaissance interiors in Florence; the walls are light grey . . .

CJ: There's no 'art-specific architecture'?

RV: We were specific in creating a special space for the Piero della Francesca panels, but even here the space is generic. A characteristic of the Early Renaissance was that rooms were quite consistent, spacially and decoratively, and we've picked up on this reference,

CJ: There's an ambiguity: on entering I would be drawn down the long, Renaissance perspective and think the sequence from the 13th century starts here – because the architecture cues it.

RV: Yes, despite the general consistency of the series of spaces we've made the central openings unusually wide and the spaces a little higher, which creates a long vista. I think this configuration will orient people; also they will be instructed in the vestibule. I think there is a mixture between didactic, chronological sequence and freedom of choice. The old palazzo that became a museum very often had this aspect.

CJ: You do have a 'both and reading' – to use one of your old phrases.

RV: One must remember the use of the building and its scale which aren't Renaissance: the whole Italian peninsula, at the time of Giotto, had about the same number of inhabitants as the crowds who will visit the museum in one year: thousands per day will have to pass by these relatively little icons.

Prince Charles and The Chameleon Building

CJ: Like it or not, the building is going to be seen as a response to Prince Charles' polemic and the debate on architecture – it's going to be sold, written about and consumed in the press as a polemical building landing in a polemical age. Do you see it reinforcing his position or counter to it?

RV: It's a perfectly sane question, but we haven't thought about it in those terms. There's always the very difficult ambiguity and tension that connects with the artist who has to do his or her things to use that expression, and connect with his or her particular view of life. At the same time the artist is a servant of the patron or the client who in turn identifies the building with the architect; at the same time, as I've said, the architect has to serve the client. So you inevitably have these fascinating tensions.

Naturally, this building has to conform to the general ideas of the trustees, the donors, the staff and Prince Charles; also it has to connect with what we feel is right. So when you work, most of the time you say – in Lou Kahn's words – 'What does the building want to be?' We also love connecting with what the place wants to be. We are not ideological, nor do we try to find a universalist solution – which, by the way, the Early Renaissance architects did. Our buildings are different wherever they are, and they are different in relation to the client. There is a balance between pleasing the client, pleasing the artist, pleasing the place and pleasing the ethos. We did not start out saying we want to please Prince Charles at all, or to servilely please the client. At the same time we get joy out of pleasing the client.

CJ: What about the literal kind of Classicism the Prince has supported, of John Simpson and Quinlan Terry? He has

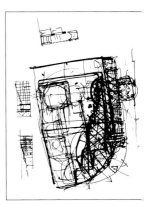

Early sketch showing the staircase idea and the view out across it: the experience of 'looking at great paintings becomes more magical after it is interrupted by the real world'.

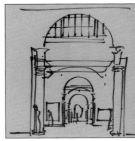

First view of galleries: the long, Renaissance perspective seen through successive arches.

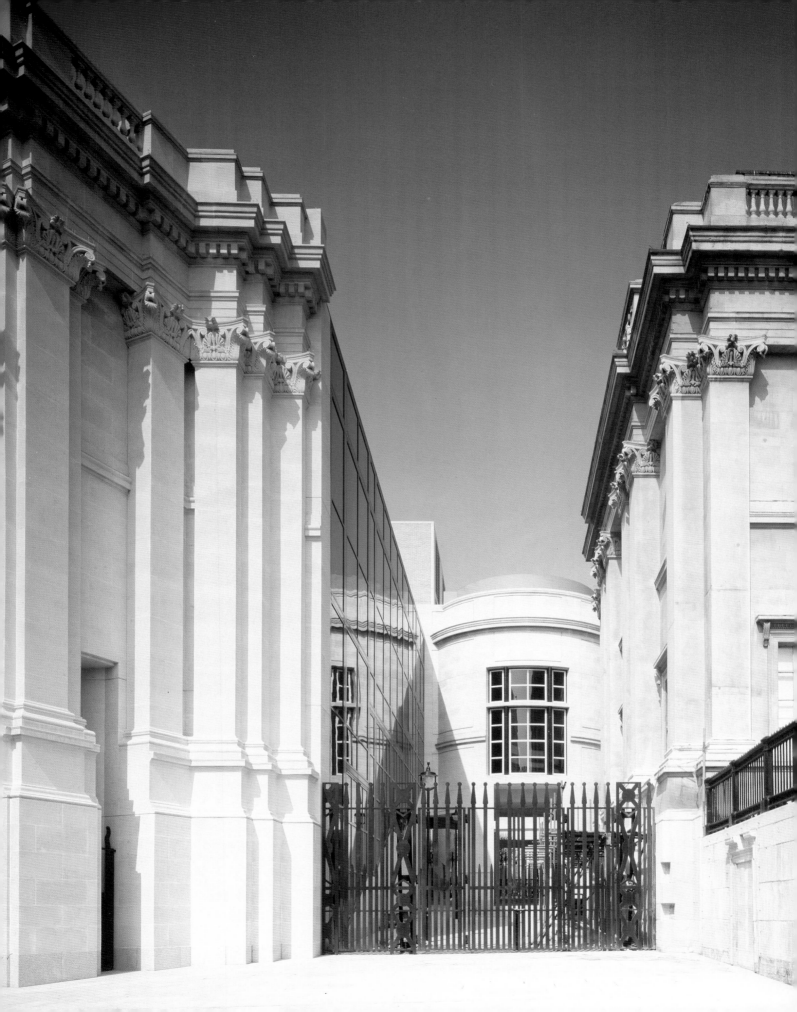

said, in his film and book *Vision of Britain*, that he has looked into the question of putting high technology behind Georgian fronts and he sees nothing problematic about that. It seems your position, and the correct Post-Modern one is that you can, technologically, do any thing you want, because there is no determinism. But it's also not very relevant to hide things behind 18th-century facades. I would argue that even though you say you're not putting forward a universalist position, to a certain extent you are: because if every building inflects towards the place, the client, the function and history and a lot of other things, then that is its own kind of universalist position. What's more, it's a better universalist position than the Prince's and the Modernists'. You are part of a tradition that's different from the Prince's.

RV: Yes, there is a kind of universality if you are going to refer to people's associations and to history: there has to be a broad range of common associations. But we really stayed away from the issue of Prince Charles' approach. As you say, a lot of that stance has evolved since the design of the building. If I were to expand on where I stand, I would say the literalist approach is not valid. As I've said, the vitality of Classical architecture in this country lies in its being Mannerist, impure, idiosyncratic, and that involves very much Inigo Jones from the beginning, Hawksmoor, and very much Soane, Greek Thomson and Wren in the churches. It involves Archer to learn from, Vanbrugh, Lutyens. I find it the most thrilling country, along with Italy and Japan.

CJ: Maybe Prince Charles isn't English enough?

RV: Just as in matters of taste it is hard to like the recent past, it is hard to know yourself.

CJ: Post-Modernism, as a tradition, has a commitment to pluralism and supporting opposite taste cultures. You also do, through your reading of Herbert Gans, and through your work. Extraordinarily, the tradition in London today is working as it is supposed to work with architects in completely opposite taste cultures designing pluralist buildings: those commercial, glitzy designers, like Ian Pollard, or the high style and serious ones like Jeremy Dixon. There are many of them in this town, even many large firms mixing high and low taste, mixing sophisticated and vulgar designs, Traditional and Modern lexicons.

They are producing a new type – what I would call the chameleon building. I suppose the first important one was Stirling's Clore Gallery in 1982, and then Jeremy Dixon's Opera House of 1987, and your building of 1986-87. But the chameleon building is now a distinctive type, particularly in London – almost creating a 'London School of Architecture'. It's surreptitious, no one set out to create it, but the developer architects are producing mixtures, you are producing hybrids and, what's more, people are reading them as mixtures and are feeling 'I enjoy that, I can understand that, it relates to me in 'my different moods'. This seems the rare case in history of cultural theory preceding action and it being proven, in a sense, correct.

In other words, the tensed field of cultural pluralism has been understood and is leading to a new intelligent eclecticism where positive meanings exist through opposition – not to the old view of cultural integration. That, it seems to me, is really the message of both your building and Post-Modernism. In the end it's different from Prince Charles, who says 'We must have an integrated culture, top down, *du haut en bas*', – and different from the Modernists, who want a populist culture *du bas en haut*; or again Le Corbusier's version which says 'We must have an élitist culture which filters down'. All of those cultural views are flawed – for us – and not working. We now live in the first culture which is beginning, like the American Constitution, to institutionalise difference and say, 'There is no way we can all live in the 18th century', or all live on the street, or live with any particular world view. What's more, intuitively, we enjoy that diversity and feel the falsity of an integrated culture. Excuse the lecture, but since you have written and built around these issues, I wanted your views. Do you feel that after 20 years of this thinking, you are winning the argument? Or do you feel, now that Post-Modernism has triumphed, these goals have been lost?

RV: Concerning so-called Post-Modernism, I am disappointed in its quality as it has evolved; on the other hand, I feel that this is a period where the extremist position (very often the least sophisticated) doesn't work. There are moments in history when the extremist position works, as there are moments of political revolution as opposed to evolution. We shouldn't try to make a revolutionary situation out of an evolutionary situation. The extremist position is ideological and simpler; whereas an evolutionary situation, naturally, is the position to project. It's much harder to write about; journalists don't like it as much, and there are fewer catchwords. It is a difficult position, you are prone to be misunderstood, where on the other hand its tolerance is appropriate in this era of vast communications, of, on the one hand, everybody coming together and knowing about everybody else, but, on the other hand, where the tribal differences are being articulated.

CJ: One of the results of the so-called Great Debate is that your 'extremists' (a very good term) have hijacked what was your 'gentle manifesto' and the debate of other tolerant people. Their extremism has hijacked it, eroded the 'vital centre' – just as it is eroded by political parties tearing at the edges. The extremists have a vested interest in demonising an enemy in order to legitimise their own counter position. Richard Rogers, Sir Norman Foster and the Modernists wanted a Prince Charles to emerge, more than anything, because a reactionary validates their avant-gardism. No *arrière-garde*, no avant-garde. Does this idiotic polarity occur in America?

RV: Yes, but in America people don't take architecture that seriously, and I hope they never do. To me it's a simplistic and boring stance . . . You have a position, but it's tolerant. You're a much happier person and better artist if you're tolerant. It's harder, but the issue is more exciting. In all the talk about style and direction, quality gets lost.

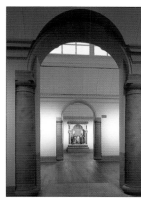

'. . . the vitality of Classical architecture in this country lies in its being Mannerist, impure, idiosyncratic'. This is an example of what I would call the chameleon building – the black glass versus the classical facade.

Diminishing perspective looking west terminating in The Incredulity of St Thomas *by Cima*

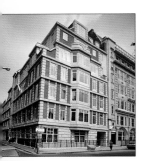

Stitching urban fabric together on three streets – Limo & Partners, 33 Golden Square (B1).

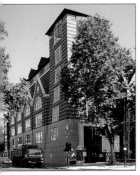

The hinge building turns and holds the corner and also here breaks up the mass into grammatical parts – DY Davies, Grove House (B8).

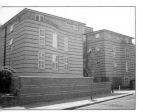

Urban infill that ties together a bend in the road – Pollard, Thomas & Edwards, Goldhawk House (B21).

Does one judge an architectural movement by its exemplars, or by its fellow-travellers? Enemies of a movement naturally take the most commercial practitioners as typical and then condemn the movement *in toto*. Defenders, by contrast, only point to the clear paragons, the Chosen Few. But perhaps the greatest focus should be on the average, the middle-of-the-road designer who has no special pretensions and who rarely achieves either much recognition or prime commissions. It is often said by historians that one learns more from a period by examining minor rather than major figures. The great poet or architect, almost by definition, is found to use the language in a heightened and abnormal way, uncharacteristic of the era as a whole. From this point of view, it is no use comparing a Mies van der Rohe with a James Stirling. Much better to contrast their followers, for they design the background building of the period. The questions then become which followers are more urbane, and able to create a professional vernacular of a high standard?

Clearly Post-Modernists have been more adept at stitching urban fabric together than the Modernists, whom they have often criticised for having destroyed it. Their work, like the Edwardians', can bend around corners, holding the street-line, then climb up or down, as necessary, to meet adjacent structures. Such urbane good manners is very evident with average Post-Modernism – what makes it civil and worthy, but not very exciting.

33 Golden Square is a good example of the genre with its red and white 'Wrenaissance' grammar that climbs around an awkward site very gracefully (B1). It is not going to inspire any young designer to leave home, but a city with a good percentage of such background buildings can count itself lucky. The same is true of the Wrenaissance housing in Flood Street, Chelsea – very urbane, moderately inventive in detail, full of crisp movement, and just a bit obvious. The inherent tendency of such architecture is to become so accommodating as to be obsequious or boring, dangers which both schemes just manage to avoid.

The Queen Anne Revival, before the Edwardian period, also produced an urbane city building but of a more eclectic kind. There are many echoes of this Free-Style Classicism in London including two corner buildings (B7, B8). The 'Westbourne' surmounts a flat layered Classicism, which is rather unsure of itself, with strong vernacular pediments (and then very weak, metal arches that look thin against the sky). 'Grove House' is a more accomplished exercise with gables and banded masonry (reminiscent of Philip Webb and Norman Shaw). But both projects are notable for their urban massing, the way they hold the corners and then break up long facades into grammatical units. All this contrasts with the mega-structures of Modernism which are continuous-endless-visual-run-on-sentences-of-no-compositional-order without hyphens, commas or full stops.

It will come as a surprise to enemies of the movement that there is much straight Post-Modernism that is well-built and 'honest' (inverted commas, as usual with Post-Modernism, indicate the *coded* nature of such concepts). Usually the approach is associated with overstatement, sophistication and irony, but there is a large segment of the tradition – stemming from the work of Aldo Rossi and Mario Botta in Europe – that adopts a straightforward attitude to building. Constructional elements are left exposed, and presented as icons of sobriety and realism. There is a latent power in this structural expressionism. The urban scheme of Jestico & Whiles on the Thames (B11), for instance, creates a taut industrial drama by contrasting vernacular volumes around an open piazza. The result is an English De Chirico – bell tower, smokestack, pitched roofs and industrial brick play off against each other in an enigmatic manner that immediately recalls Metaphysical Painting and Magic Realism.

Richard Reid, also on the Thames (A33), plays it very straight and vernacular with the housing which syncopates its way around a flat stretch of water – a conceptual piazza. Here the intersecting of complex rhythms is frantically Baroque, while the surfaces are understated vernacular, and the contrast between these two genres very pleasing. One of the most satisfying examples of similar straightforwardness is Goldhawk House on Goldhawk Road in West London (B21), an infill block that very subtly ties together a slight bend in the road and then symbolises the idea with gentle curves. The eclecticism is understated – the banded masonry, the square Rossian windows, and the roof-massing reminiscent of early Frank Lloyd Wright. But what finally convinces one about this ingenious piece of urbanism is its no-nonsense handling of very old ideas and materials. This is perennial architecture (or what the Traditionalists would call 'timeless' were it not Post-Modern).

There is a counter-tradition even within this compact genre of civil and worthy urbanism: Post-Modern Baroque. Much more worldly and commercial than the Rossian-inspired design, it adapts old motifs to new purposes: Baroque rhythms, diagonals, facets, triangular windows and layered ornament. Here the Post-Modern hybridisation is most apparent: today's technologies of glass, steel and concrete produce new proportions and new feelings using the old Baroque repertoire. Invention flows inevitably from such simple conjunctions, for instance from having to detail stone in glass. Hybridisation thus becomes highly visual, and symbolic of the oxymoron 'past/present'. 'Brookmount House' on Chandos Place (B26) has giant triangular windows on the first floor, surmounted by two floors of Y-fronted windows and a double attic. Polychromatic brick underscores the window rhythms and basic tripartition. The building can thus play a background role and hold the street-line, while still creating new syncopations and surface punctuations.

DY Davies, in Holborn, has produced a Mannerist hybrid which layers so many references – face, body, church, keystones, arches, banded concrete – that one can spend hours decoding the superimposed readings (B27). Modernists, of course, hate this sort of complexity, and only provide one or two readings in their univalent facades – orders which are consumed at a glance. Paradoxically they accuse Davies' sort of building of pandering to easy visual consumption – when the six visual layers are not at all obvious and take a certain creative imagination to unravel.

On Enford Street and Marylebone Road, Hamilton Associates (B30) create a Baroque syncopation not only between the usual diagonals and rectangles, but also be-tween polished granite and glass, grey and white zones, and blue and black elements. The multiple readings are a delight in a building which seems at first glance just another massive groundscraper. When one turns the corner of Enford Street and sees how the massing and grammar are transformed into the low-scaled Georgian, one appreciates how much the lessons of urbanity and eclecticism have been taken up in mainstream practice. Such buildings vindicate the idea of a Post-Modern tradition extending not only from the top down – *du haut en bas* – but from commerce up.

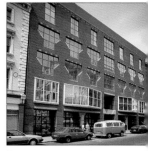

Straightforward industrial PM – Jestico and Whiles, Burrell's Wharf, (B11).

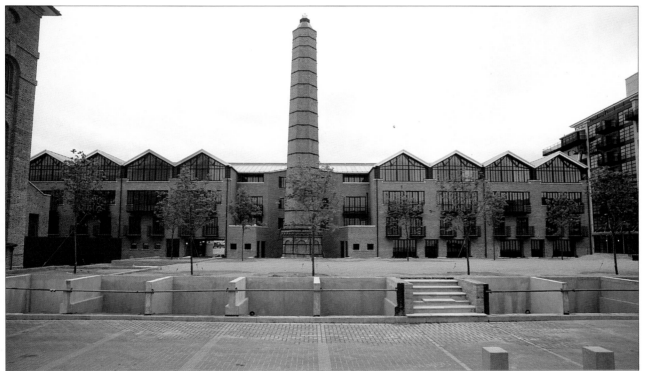

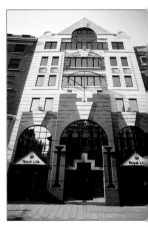

Baroque syncopations, Y-shapes and V-form windows – Rock Townsend, Brookmount House (B26).

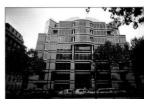

Multiple readings are layered – DY Davies, Spec Office (B27).

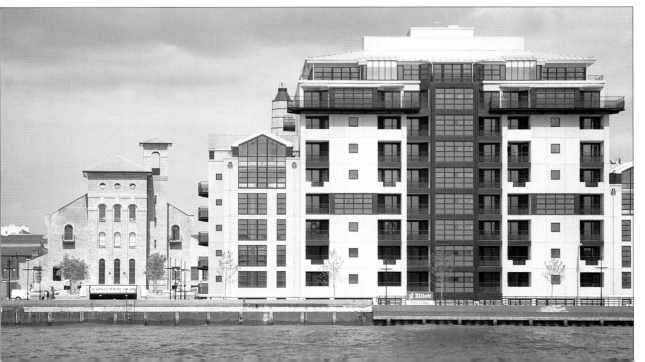

Baroque Oppositions, movement of profile and diagonal corner towers – Hamilton Associates, 151 Marylebone Road (B30).

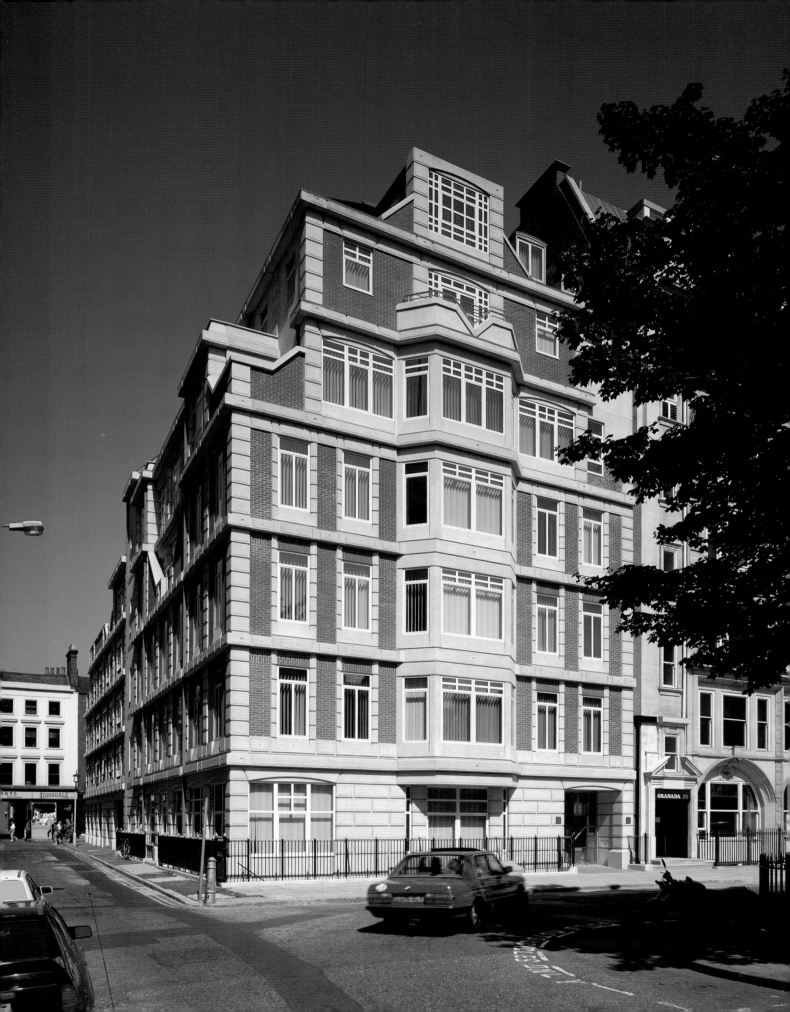

33 URBANE POST-MODERN BUILDINGS

B1 LIMO AND PARTNERS, 33 Golden Square W1, 1989. No doubt Modernists would claim it a fussy building, but look how well it mediates between two different scales – the sober rhythms of Beak Street and the urbanity of Golden Square. Many small-scaled elements in light concrete break up the bulk – quoins, cuts, flares, fillets, small round voids, projecting bays and the ubiquitous V-forms. The way the building steps back and handles three different street conditions makes up for the rather predictable ornament.

B2 THE MACDONALD PRICE PARTNERSHIP, 56-64 Flood Street, Chelsea SW3, 1986-88. 10 town houses form a cluster of subtle ABA rhythms and an opposition between red brick and cream stone (actually cast stone). Large dividing walls, ending in pillars, separate each front garden. Steel railings with circular Mackintoshian capitals, painted black, enclose the garage areas.

B3 JOHN MELVIN AND PARTNERS, Mercer's Place, Brook Green W6, 1984. The architect cites Norman Shaw as a precedent for his version of the Queen Anne Revival – ruddy brick, white trim, playing a Classical game with Modern counters – and one can see what he means. The windows have the large, flat abstract design so redolent of the 60s, while chimneys, arches and overhanging eaves recall the hybrid styles of the 1880s and 1890s. Other touches recall Lutyens, such as the chequer-pattern and nicely exaggerated chimney stacks. It's all very convincing and civilised.

The architect writes:

'Post-Modern Classicism . . . At Essex Road the influence of Norman Shaw is pronounced. The architecture fully acknowledges Modernism with its constructional imperatives such as the extensive use of precast concrete, but it also attempts to extend the language and embrace traditional architecture. Like Shaw, I am seeking to draw upon not just the 17th-century English Baroque, but an earlier nascent Classicism where the Tudor and Jacobean were evolving into it. The strongly articulated service towers either side of the entrance doors have their parallel in the Tudor gate-houses of the Cambridge colleges or pre-Wren Hampton Court. These service towers and lift shafts reinforce this image as they punctuate the skyline. Pierced balustrades at parapet level provide a degree of layering and enhance the silhouette, acknowledging the special quality of English light. The use of red brick to contrast with the white precast con-

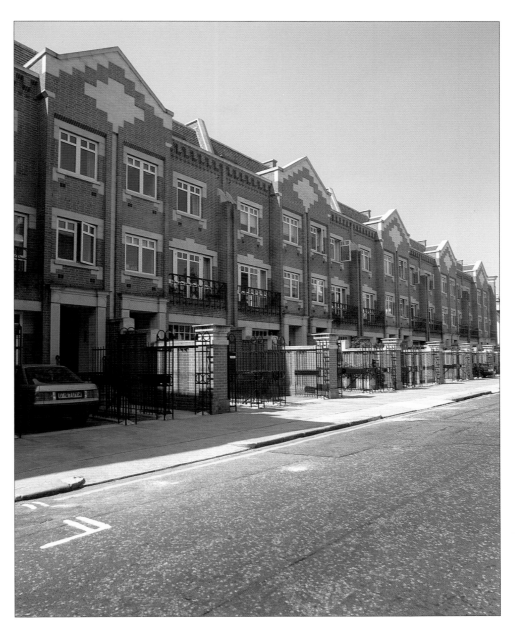

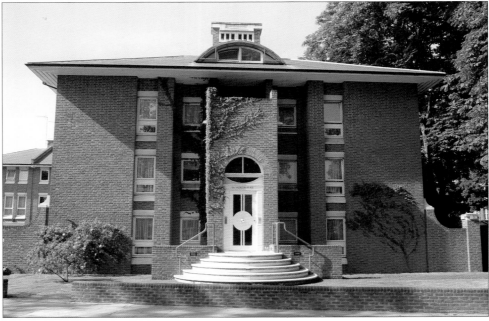

crete makes obvious reference to Tudor architecture as does the chequerboard pattern. This pattern runs through the design like a leitmotif, but it is treated in a thoroughgoing Modernist way – serial and machine-made. It occurs not just in the service towers, which can be read as giant Orders, but is repeated around lunettes over the stairwells and around the door cases.

I have attempted to broaden the usual frame of Post-Modern Classical reference, beyond the Neo-Classical and Palladian, by alluding to the more native Artisan Mannerism and the English Baroque. The result is a modern solution to a modern programme without the usual recourse to pastiche or parody.

John Melvin

B4 *JOHN MELVIN AND PARTNERS, Sheltered Housing, Essex Road N1, in construction 1990.*

B5 *JOHN MELVIN AND PARTNERS, Sheltered Housing and Group Practice surgery, Mitchison Road N1, in construction 1990.*

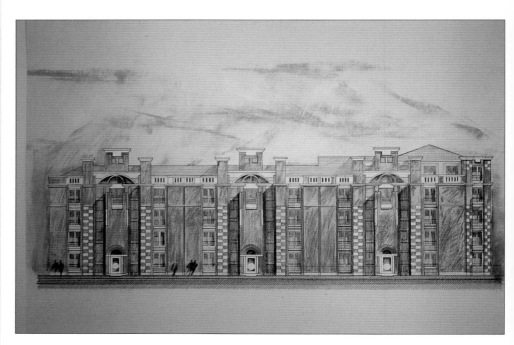

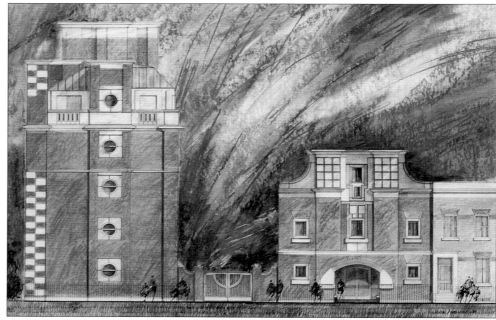

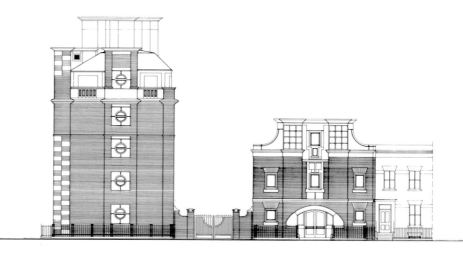

B6 *COVELL, MATTHEWS, WHEATLEY, Trinity Court, Bishops Bridge Road, London W2, 1987. Very civilised housing which holds the street-line to which it presents a sober exterior. A rusticated base, with the ubiquitous Rossian windows, is surmounted by a brick middle, with bands, and then long, overhanging eves à la Wright. Occasional High-Tech elements are picked out in dark blood red, or blue. The urbanity of the image is reminiscent of New York and Berlin.*

B7 *DOUGLAS PASKIN ASSOCIATES, The Westbourne, 118 Westbourne Grove W11, 1988. This corner building of 48 flats and 6 penthouses holds strong vernacular pediments on a slightly unsure, flat, layered, Classical base; but unfortunately it tops the Free-Style Classicism with weak metal arches. A pleasant sheltered courtyard is on the inside of the perimeter block.*

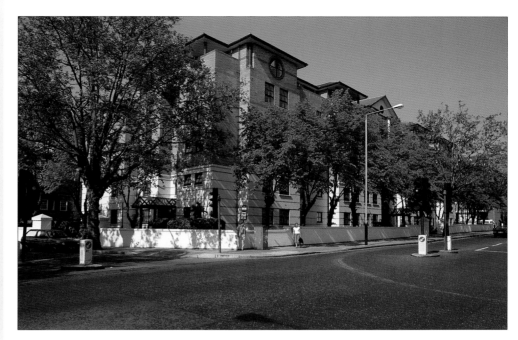

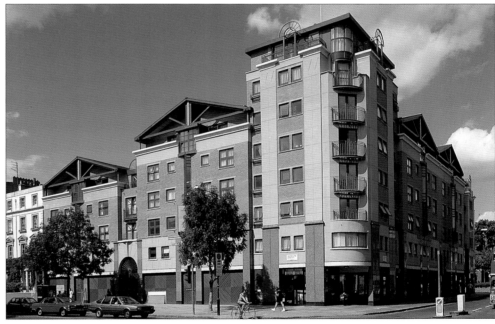

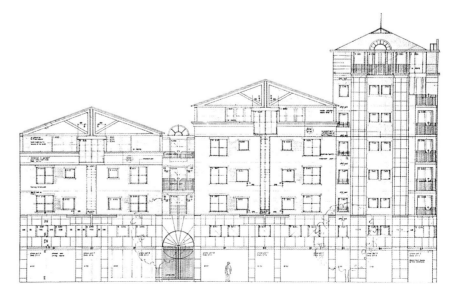

B8 DY DAVIES, *Grove House, 248 Marylebone Road NW1, 1989, offices. Free-Style Classical redevelopment, using vestiges of Marylebone Grammar School, breaks the long facade into grammatical units with gables and banded masonry à la Philip Webb. Part of an overall development of two office buildings and a block of flats, this Neo-Queen Anne Revival building makes urbane good sense.*

B9 WILLIAM WHITFIELD, *Richmond House, office infill, 79 Whitehall W1, 1986-88. Four small and one clustered tower in yellow brick and stone take up the colours of the buildings on either side, but change the style from Neo-Classical to Post-Modern Gothick. The banded 'zebra-look' is supposed to relate to Norman Shaw's nearby Old Scotland Yard, but that is a russet Wrenaissance building, not a cream and yellow custard. The overall massing can only be described as a muscle-bound interpretation of oriel windows, bay rhythms and towers – a Neo-Perpendicular medieval church married to a Neo-Brutalist office. What does this symbolism say about the occupant, the Department of Health?*

B10 DAVID QUIGLEY, *Hopewell Yard, 25 Hopewell Street, Camberwell SE5, 1988-90. Housing, offices and light industrial premises unified in a block which holds the street lines and creates an active interior courtyard. Urban polychromy of red, yellow and blue brick sets up optical vibrations, while flashes of white stucco hold anthropomorphic shapes – including a long-nosed horse.*

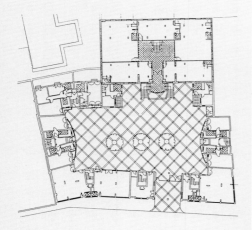

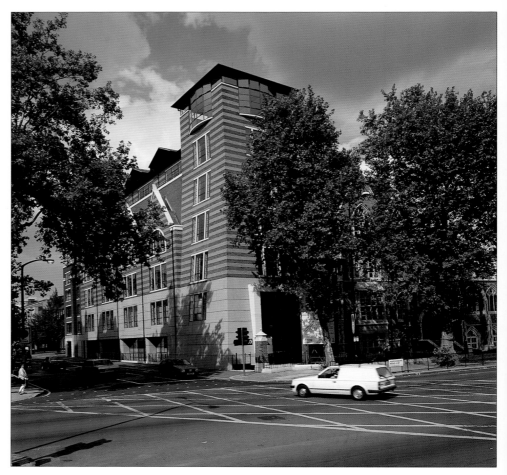

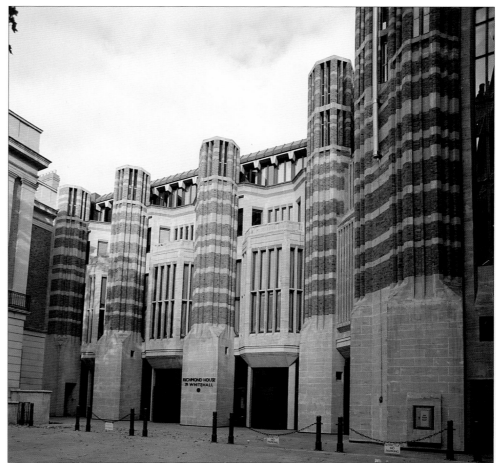

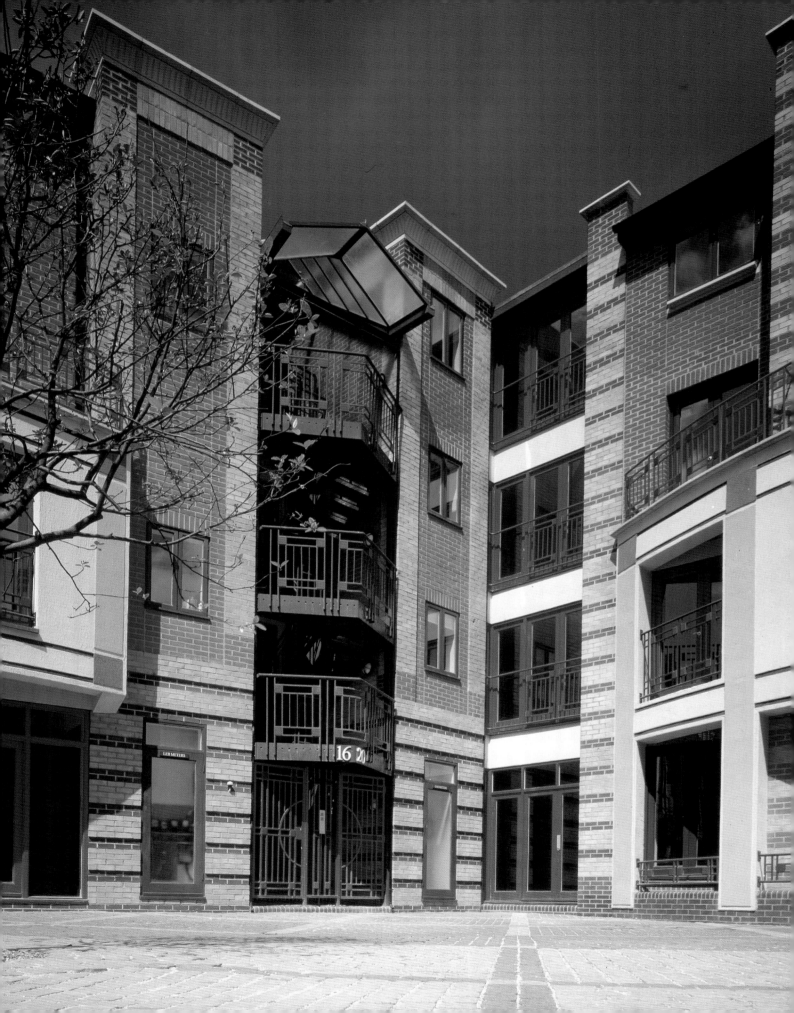

B11 *JESTICO AND WHILES, Burrell's Wharf, 262 Westferry Road, Isle of Dogs E14, 1990. Phase 1: 152 apartments, leisure centre, retail; Phase 2: 178 apartments, 10 business units, 8 shops – Open programme.* As Stephanie Williams writes, this group, formerly the Millwall Ironworks, is the only historically interesting group of industrial buildings on the Isle of Dogs comparable to the great warehousing complexes on the South Bank of the river. Laid out in 1836 by William Fairbairn, pioneer of structural ironwork and successful Manchester shipbuilder, it was the first purpose-built shipyard in England. The old offices originally built by Cubitt are being repaired to stop further deterioration, while the rather Italianate Central Plate House will soon be a leisure centre. The great chimney, with its original corset of iron supports now serves as a flue for heating. Two new blocks of 80 flats, each of concrete slab construction with storey-height pre-cast wall panels make much use of steel detailing. River views and the industrial drama of contrasting volumes combine to produce an English De Chirico.

B12 *RICHARD JUPP, Free Trade Wharf, The Highway, Shadwell E1, 1988.* Straightforward structural expressionism in the conversion of two 1795 East India Co warehouses into a small neighbourhood grouping around the original York stone paved courtyard. The symmetrical wings focus on the Thames with all the force of a bowling alley, or at least one-point perspective which one cannot avoid. Low four-storey buildings contain six apartments, a small hotel, leisure facilities and arcades of shops.

B13 *KIT ALLSOPP ARCHITECTS, Docklands Sailing Centre, Kingsbridge, Millwall Dock E14, 1989.* Ubiquitous 'Wharfism' – portholes, wood decks, exaggerated timber, big-boat scale.

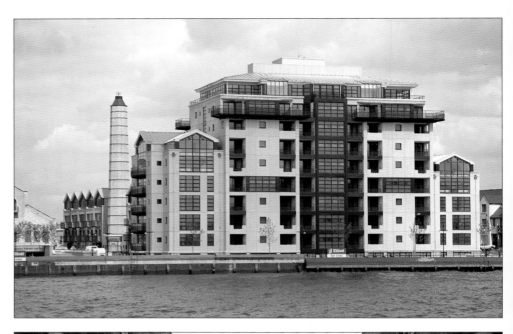

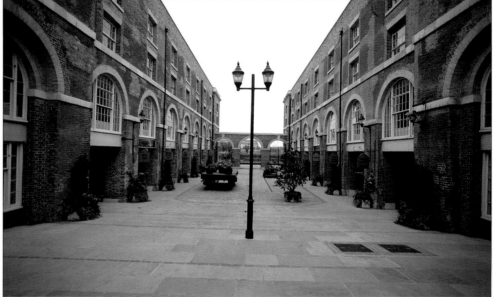

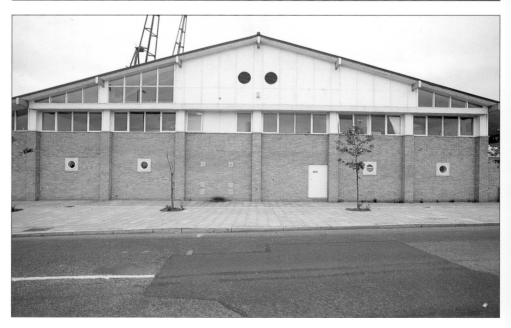

B14 STOUT AND LITCHFIELD, *West Ferry Road and Wynan Road E14, 1988. As Stephanie Williams points out, these narrow terrace houses are the largest self-build housing development in UK, created under the direction of Dr Michael Barraclough. Is this what people really want when they build their own houses? Given the amount of designers, the aesthetic consistency and repetition are surprising: the timber detailing, white bricks, slate roofs are like Dr Barraclough's own house down river – solid, straightforward vernacular at its best. The scheme received a* Times/*RIBA Community Enterprise Award in 1988.*

B15 KJAER AND RICHTER, *Greenland Passage, South Sea Street, off Redriff Road SE16, 1989. Very pleasing sober symmetries and details define an urbane realm on the garden side. 152 flats and townhouses, in Portland stone and pale yellow Danish brick, form regular urban spaces – rectangles, semicircles, squares. Note the occasional Rossian touch of the square sash window or, by the street entrance, the strong arch set against the curve of the stairs and columns. The shapes and composition have a taut, tough rationality – is this the Danish version of the Mediterranean tradition? In any case the mixture of nine-storey blocks, three-storey houses and ingeniously interlocking space shows an urbanist at work.*

B16 SHEPPARD ROBSON, *Montpelier House, 106-110 Brompton Road SW3 1983. These offices, with houses hidden behind, take up the Pont Street Dutch vernacular nearby and make this a pretext for some very abstract brick gables – machined brick laid in five different ornamental patterns. The abstraction is intensified by the flat planes of glass and use of only two materials. Note the Greek Cross pattern at the top, which creates little stub finials.*

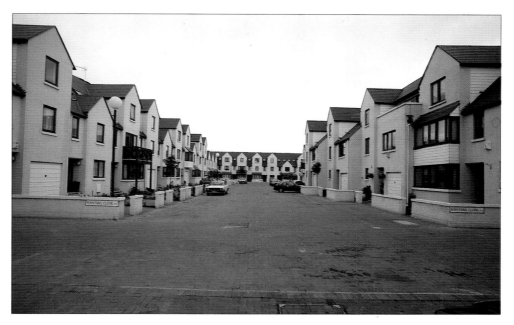

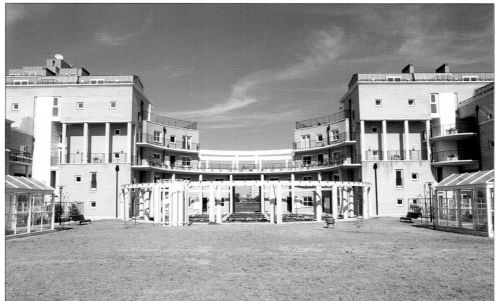

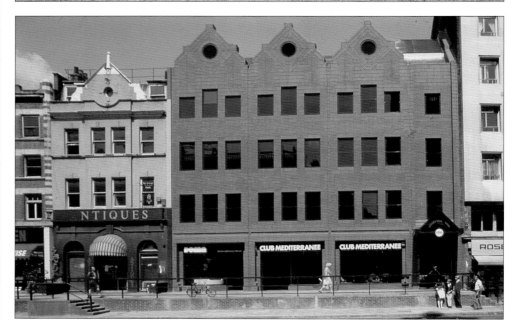

B17 CHASSAY WRIGHT ARCHITECTS, *Bridge Wharf, Caledonian Road and Regents Canal, Kings Cross N1, 1986-88. This series of 21 'live/work' units takes its abstracted arches, paired windows, rectangular volumes and Ibstock golden russet brickwork from the nearby Kings Cross Terminal Building by Thomas Cubbitt. To this are added the ubiquitous Post-Modern V-windows and exaggerated skylights (visible on the canal side). Understated historical precedents are also well hidden in the overall massing – the rendered triumphal arch, the curved, brick apse – very effective allusions, the more so for being so ambiguous. Most of the units have ended up being sold to advertisers, public relations companies, computer firms, for example, but they can still be lived in.*

B18 CHASSAY WRIGHT ARCHITECTS, *Coutts Crescent, 12-23 St Albans Road, Highgate NW5, 1989. This is one of the best examples of the terrace housing revival in its new form (for others see MacCormac's Shadwell Basin, etc A35, A36). Nine houses form a slightly curved crescent that ends in two pavilion houses – with their squat colonnades forming entrance loggias. The uniform sobriety of the terrace formula is created by the ubiquitous square Rossian windows on the first floor and the steady rhythm of banded brick piers below – a rhythm however which is gently syncopated. At either end two 'Jencksianas' – semi-circular pediments plus staggers focus the axis, while a very understated central focus to the front is created by a squared circular window. All in all the sequence of space – semi-public, semi-private, private, private garden – is well handled by this perennial formula, and the uniformity is subtly broken by the alternations of grey and cream.*

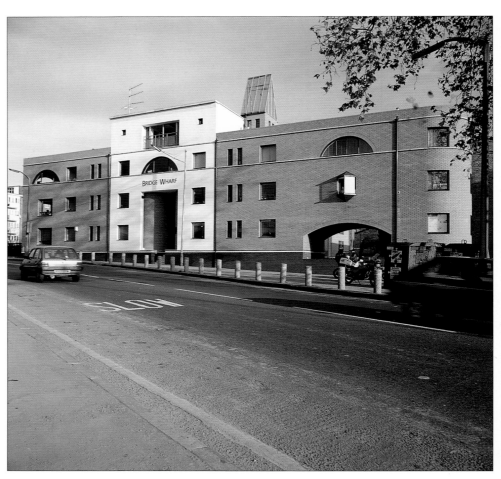

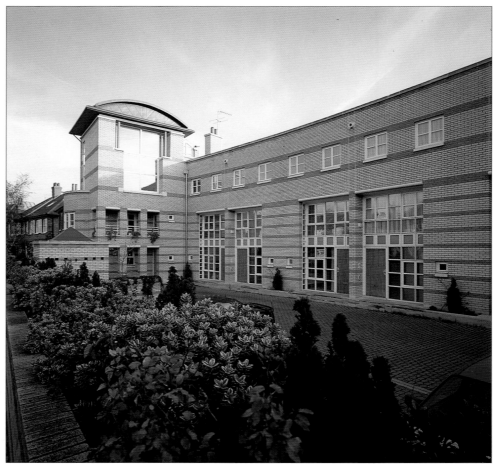

B19 CHASSAY ARCHITECTS, *The Fitzpatrick Building, York Way and Vale Royal, Kings Cross N1, 1988-91. Another corner building with a round 'hinge' (like Farrell's buildings A8, A10) which here steps up to the all important glazed oval cylinder that holds the client's offices. This is given extra punch with a ruddy [russet] brown flare and the contrast with a green penthouse. A green granite base of the long part of the L-block is surmounted by a neutral wall of buff-coloured birch, steel and glass – early Modernism married to the Renaissance. The overall mass seems to plough through the troubled waters of Kings Cross like a long oil tanker.*

B20 CHASSAY ARCHITECTS, *Town Hall, Isle of Dogs E14, 1988-91. Again early Modern marries the Renaissance with the former quite appropriately containing the Council offices and the latter suitably holding the Council Chamber. Docklands nautical versus democratic Classical, ship versus rotunda, rather obvious contrasts which are given subtle twists within and without. Note again the ubiquitous Gravesian 'flare' similar to Richard Reid's Civic Centre (A32).*

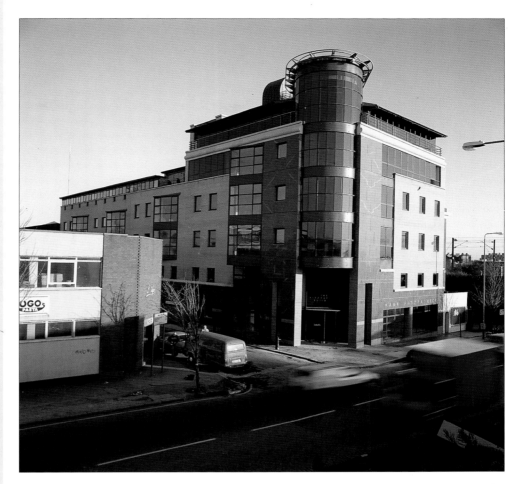

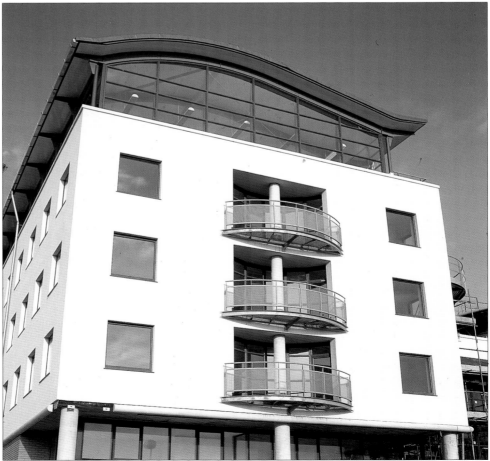

B21 *POLLARD, THOMAS AND EDWARDS,*
Goldhawk House, 191 Goldhawk Road W3,
1989. 21-bedroom sheltered flats for the
elderly with common room and garden.
Semicircular, high-tech pediment over the
entrance focuses the axis between the slightly
curved bays on either end which subtly
reflect a slight bend in the road. These tie
the two different lines of adjacent buildings
and resolve them into a central, indented
bay. Pseudo sash windows, à la Rossi, and
an early Frank Lloyd Wright cornice give
this modest urban infill a wide reference.

B22 *ROBSHAW RICHMOND, Bricklayers*
Arms Depot, Mandela Way, SE1, 1990. A
continuous curved I-beam, used as an en-
tablature, unites banded brick pavilions with
recessed horizontal coursing – offices –
which are placed in front of simple rectangles
of warehouse space. The Post-Modern dou-
ble-coding creates an interesting oppositional
rhythm by being as logical and straightfor-
ward as possible.

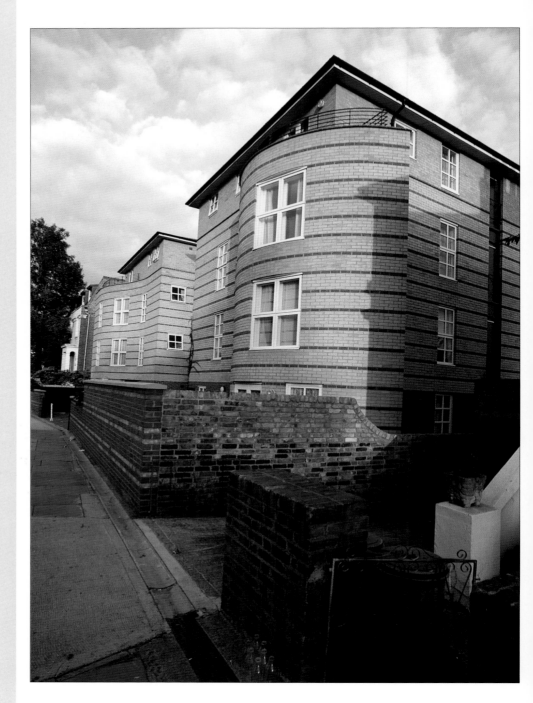

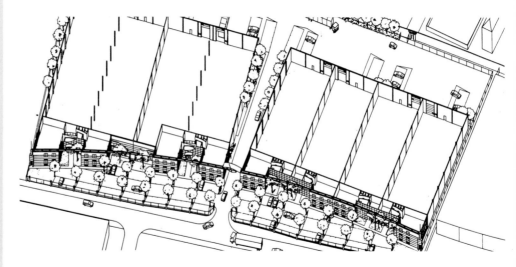

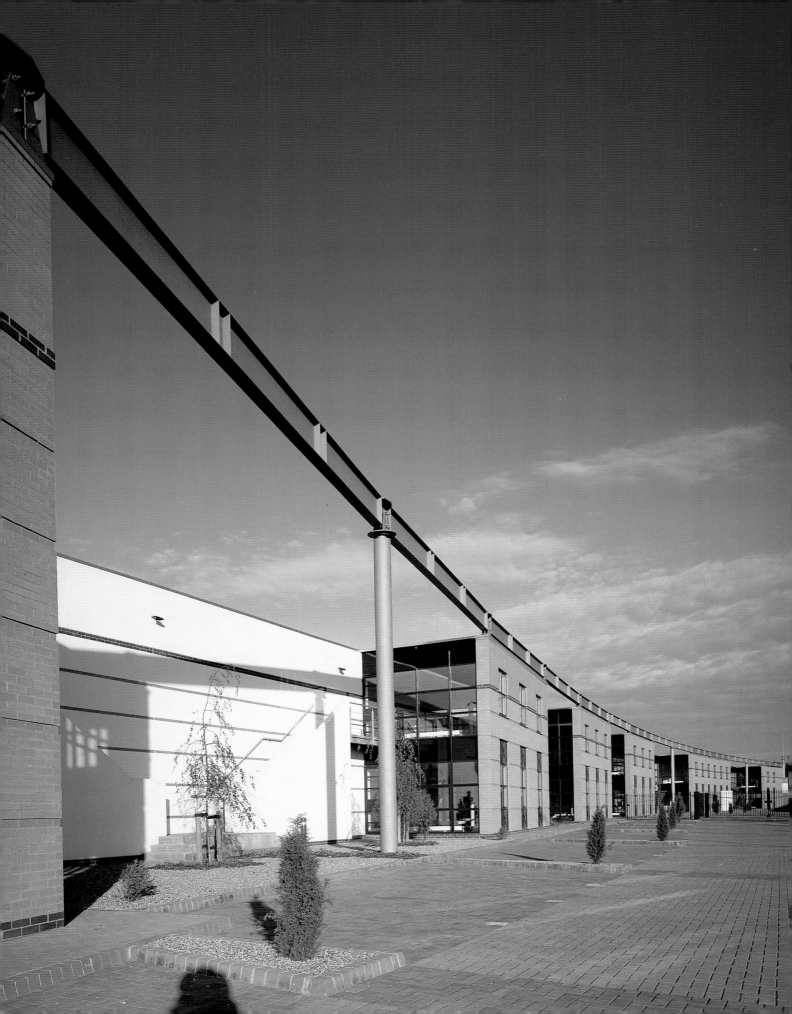

B23 JAMES GORST, Gibson House, Islington N1, 1987. An exceptional culmination of a Georgian terrace which transforms the Neo-Classical language in subtle ways starting with the tapered 'Egyptian' light-house pylons at the entrance, continuing up to the cantilevered horizontals of the balconies and doors and then to the 'attic' floor treated as a cross between early Wright and Egyptian. The proportional relationship of brick to stucco and twin pavilion to set back is strong, obvious and sensible. This is urbane Post-Modernism in its most civil mode.

B24 COLQUHOUN MILLER AND PARTNERS, Housing, Church Crescent E9, 1984. Four to eight person houses are placed like tense little boxes on a slightly curved street. Their taut quality is reinforced by the low hipped roofs and the austere symmetrical shapes organised with a tight economy. Window voids are punched into the plane surfaces to create well-proportioned primary forms.

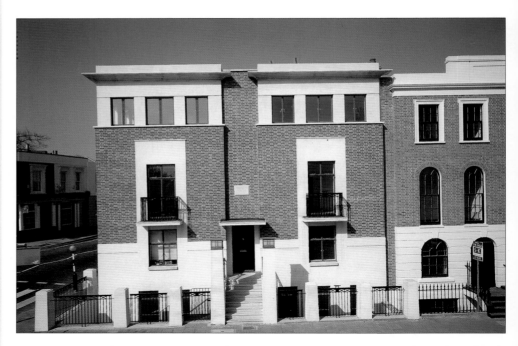

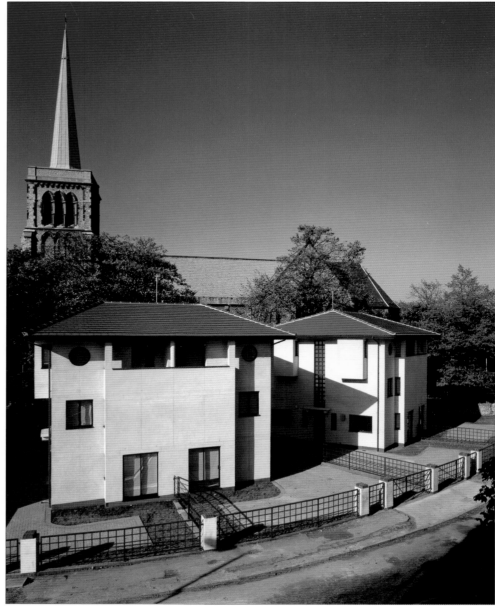

B25 *COLQUHOUN MILLER AND PART-NERS, Housing, Albion Drive, Shrubland Road, Brownlaw Road E8, 1984. The single family terrace house form, broken up into flats of different size, is a formula that Jeremy Dixon (A3) and others use, as here, to fit in with a 19th-century street architecture and give a familiar small-scaled pattern to new social realities. Very simple rhythms – often pairs of pairs – create interesting symmetries within symmetries. The Post-Modern Classicism of London stock brick above a rusticated base surrounds a shared giant door with ubiquitous Rossian windows.*

B26 *ROCK TOWNSEND, Brookmount House, 62-65 Chandos Place WC2, 1982-84. Tripartite rhythms of giant triangular and Y-fronted windows are echoed by polychromatic brick ornamentation. The splayed form of the large bay window in the* piano nobile *is taken up in the concrete capitals of the ground floor and the diagonals of the third and fourth floors, giving unity to this strange mixture of Baroque and vernacular.*

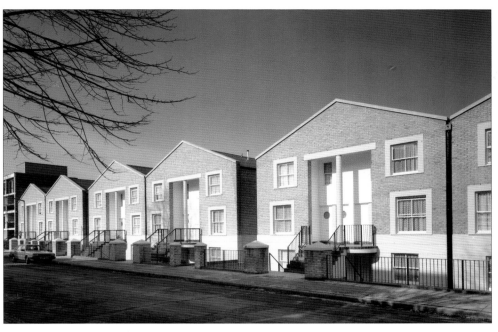

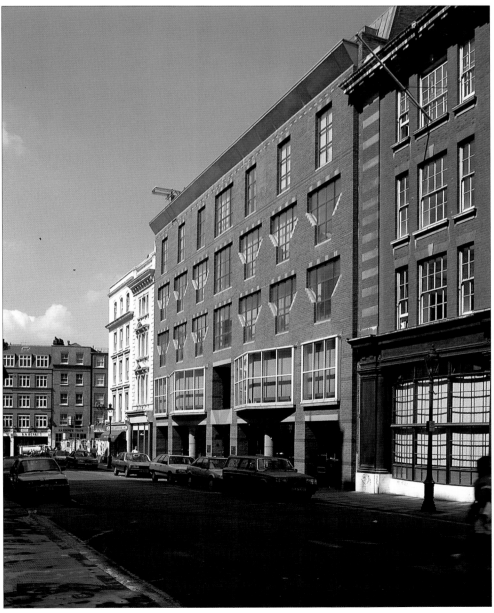

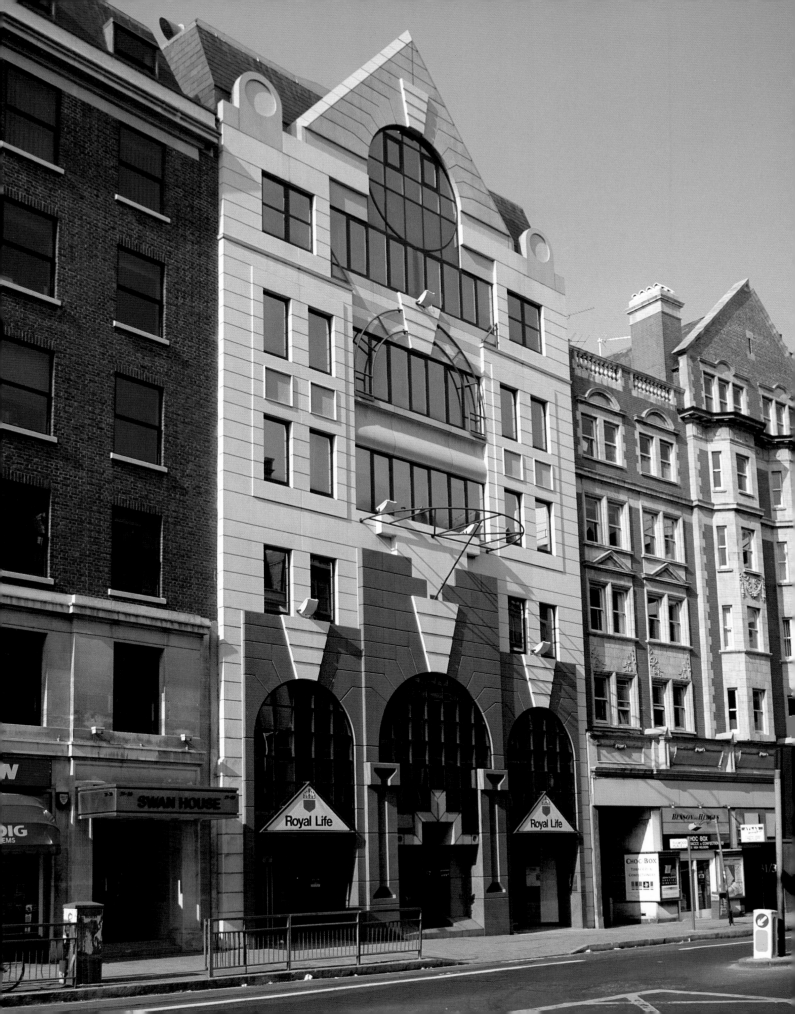

B27 *DY DAVIES, Spec Office, 34-36 High Holborn WC1, 1986-88. This hybrid design incorporates references to the face, body, church, keystones, arches, banded concrete, etc, and layers them in a very shallow, intense space. It's the welcome antithesis of the dumb office block with only one reading.*

B28 *DAMOND LOCK GRABOWSKI PART-NERS, King's Walk Shopping Mall, 122 King's Road, Chelsea SW3, 1986-88. A brick, Rossian facade is cracked open to invite shoppers into an interior curved atrium surrounded by glistening King's Road boutiques and hot spots. The architecture, with its flash exuberance and collision between High-Tech and Classicism, captures this world quite well. One of the great solecisms of architectural grammar is carried through with disarming panache: the semi-circular canopy placed above round columns. Alberti said 'Never!'; but here the disjunction of grammars is mediated by a broken truss. The 'palazzo' facade is layered like a geode; atrium, bridge, elevator and staircase leap about like players in the old Constructivist drama* The Man Who Was Thursday.

B29 *BRIAN TAGGART, House, 71 Warwick Road and corner of Pembroke Gardens W8, 1990. This large house contrasts a central cylindrical bay with an octagonal corner bay, and a general white grammar with various aluminium geometries. The roof is full of a subtle movement which Vanbrugh would have liked.*

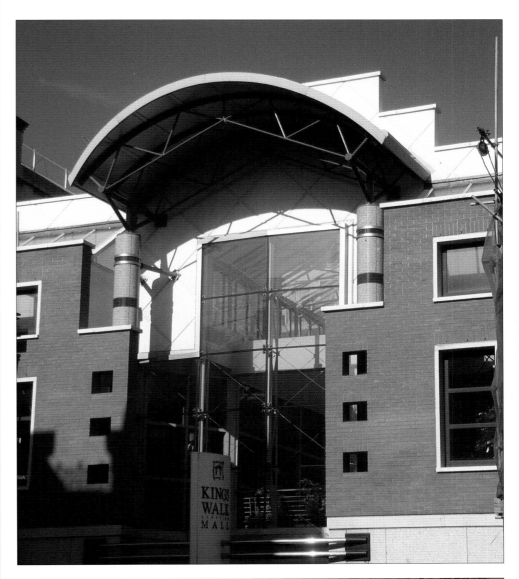

B30 *HAMILTON ASSOCIATES, job architect, Izslot Malden, 151 Marylebone Road and Enford Street W1, 1989-90. High-Tech Baroque splays its corner towers on the diagonal like a Borromini church made from chunky metal and flat stone. At first glance this office building looks crude, yet subtle effects are produced as it lowers its bulk and changes grammar to accommodate the Georgian of Enford Street. Metal and stone, silver and black, solid and void are syncopated and reversed across the facade to give its undulations more movement. The five-bay rhythm of the Marylebone facade is punctuated by major reversals between light grey granite, dark granite, metal and glass. Little pyramidal tops and slight curves lessen the monolithic heaviness: this 'skylump' is made less lumpy by articulations.*

B31 *MIKE TRICKETT, ROLFE JUDD GROUP, Central Capital, 4 Park Place W1, 1986-88. This clever urban office infill unites two street-levels with a connecting stair, balancing a slight incline of the road to the left with the asymmetrical symmetry of the loggia to the right. Post-Modern Doric columns diminish slightly against an undulating facade of white concrete, banded with horizontal grooves of incised fillet ornament, that cuts through the top third of the windows.*

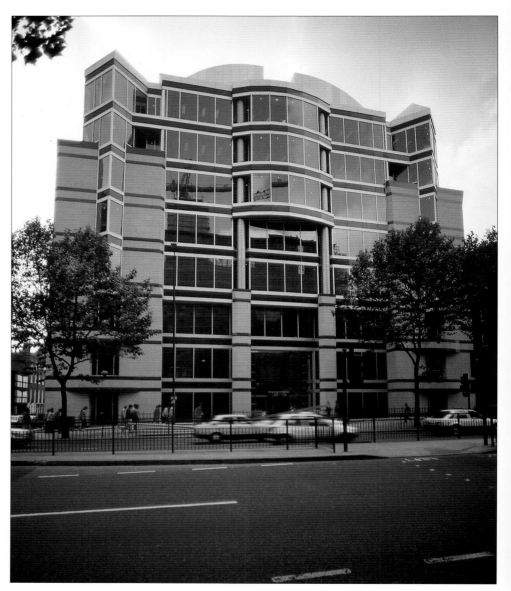

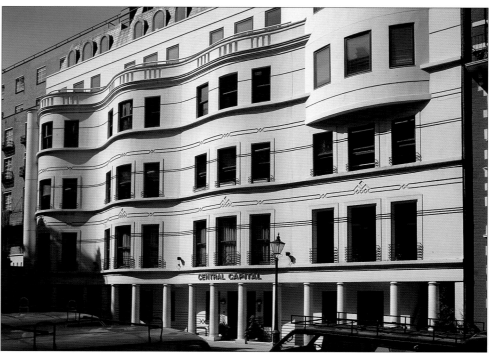

B32 BUILDING DESIGN PARTNERSHIP, Ealing Centre, Ealing Broadway W5, 1985. The nearly Neo-Gothic town hall is a pretext for an eclectic Neo-Queen Anne Revival – 'playing a Classical game with Gothic counters' – or is it the other way around? In any case this monolithic shopping mall, office and sports centre is subtracted of its usual crude formless bulk, and given brick bay rhythms, oriel windows, pediments and brooding roof-forms.

B33 TED LEVY BENJAMIN & PARTNERS (now ARCHITECTURAL DESIGN ASSOCIATES), Designing Partner Ike Horvitch, 100 Avenue Road NW3, 1983-85. This building has an urban quality which gives presence to an otherwise chaotic Swiss Cottage 'racetrack'. Six-storey, basically Classical, symmetrical office building (with two restaurants on the ground floor) organised on a horizontal white grid of travertine marble with a frame of blood red powdered aluminium, which gives slight asymmetrical touches when used as an interior window. The red frame breaks into the white grid to give further syncopation to the two rhythms, and dark grey circles punctuate the main cross-lines as if to underline the markings on an original drawing. The omnipresent rectangular geometry is further modified by the stepped echelons of the overall mass which comes towards the street as the building descends.

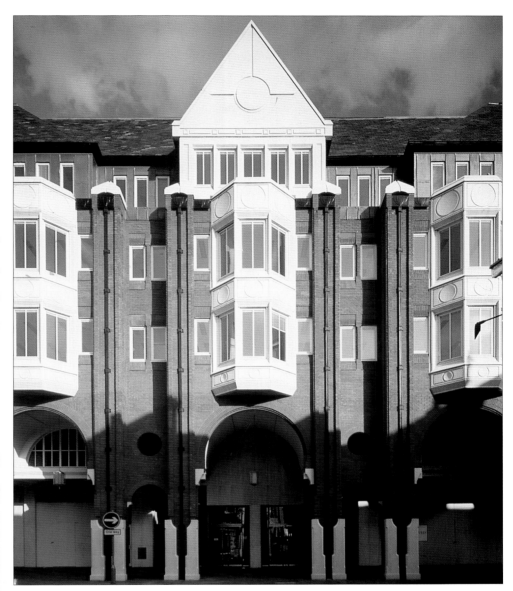

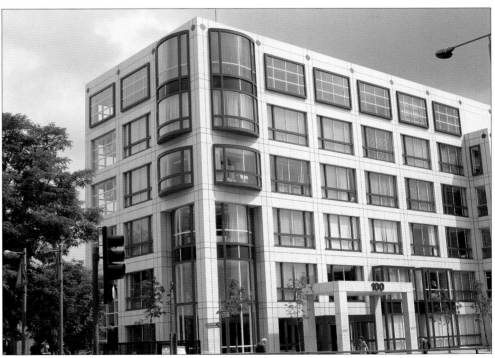

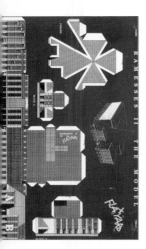

Parody and pastiche of high culture sources from Nouvel, Pei and Egypt, applied to another shed building, Ian Pollard's Ramesses II (model kit).

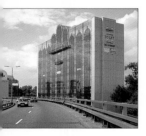

Post-Modernisation of a slab block improves acoustics, interior comfort and leaves the eye-strain of the kind of architecture meant to be perceived at 40 mph – Covell Matthews Wheatley, Vantage West on the M4 overpass (C19).

The 1980s, the Thatcher and Reagan Era as it is known to pessimists, no doubt had its dark and excessively commercial side. The unacceptable facade of capitalism was exploited by Modernists and Post-Modernists alike, although the latter only receive credit for being so venal. Vulgarity, it seems, is only evident when it is overstated. Yet if it is true Modernists were just as opportunistic as other architects, it is also a fact that Post-Modernists were quicker to embrace, and more adept at creating, the kitsch, commercial style. Partly this was due to their belief in rhetoric, ornament and polychromy, and partly it was due to their pluralism; the conviction that all tastes matter and that high and low taste-cultures can be mixed.

High culture architects such as Terry Farrell and Piers Gough will occasionally use low culture motifs and themes: thus their work always has a dose of healthy vulgarity about it. But it is really Ian Pollard who has turned high culture into low – and almost back again – with his inventive rip-offs of James Stirling, Richard Rogers, Philip Johnson and Egyptian civilisation. In his eclecticism Pollard is *the* commercial counterpart of Stirling, employing the same conflictive logic and wit. The only difference is education, taste and sensibility; a big 'only' for most people. Yet this should not obscure the creative pluralism which underlies Pollard's work.

For the Sainsbury Homebase off Cromwell Road, he decorates the shed with Stirling's Stuttgart to one side and Imperial Egyptian to the other, placing several zig-zag, architectural cut-lines in between (C1). These accentuate the oppositions of style and meaning and underline the fact that all the images are merely veneers applied to a steel frame. The thin peels and juxtapositions are Stirlingesque and essentially Post-Modern: they create an ornament which is both didactic and amusing, decoration which tells you it is a sign of a sign.

Inevitably, Sainsbury's wanted their Homebase to be a respectable monument, a discrete advertisement and a logo all at once – probably something impossible to achieve without contradiction. So when faced with the explicit historical reference, they whitewashed out some of the Egyptian iconography (inadvertently leaving it even more exotic). Thus embarrassment has conspired to create some very pleasing ambiguities which no one has intended – for instance the transformation of polychromatic Egyptian gods and goddesses into black and white realism. I'm sure this odd sequence is just what the shopper wants to see as he or she heads from the parking lot to the shed – the enigmatic changing of frogs into princes, or consumer durables into Homebase icons. With this building Pollard emerged as the noble savage of kitsch, the heroic and shameless psychoanalyst of the contradictory motives which boil in every shopper's heart.

Next door to Homebase and under construction is *Ramesses II*, an amalgam of IM Pei's glass pyramid, Jean Nouvel's camera-lens windows and a glass version of the temples at Abu Simbel. The results will be deplored by the professional press and Pollard will take over the role, from Robert Stern, as the most Sincerely Hated Architect At Work (although in private many architects will grant his courage and inventiveness).

For the Marco Polo House, and *The Observer*, he has produced a Pop-Classical facade to cover an open plan, high-tech interior (C2). The contradictions extend beyond style to include differences of scale, detail and mood. Where the exterior is huge and related to the adjacent gasometer and Battersea Power Station (both scaleless Pop structures in their way), the inside is soft, broken up in detail and space, and even quite friendly. Philip Johnson's broken pediment towers over the canted, ultra-smooth legs of the building – which look as if they have elephantiasis – while Richard Rogers' Lloyds becomes the pretext for making a pretty interior landscape.

If in kitsch nothing succeeds like excess, then Pollard's buildings get high pass marks. They are redeemable as grotesques, as frightening schlock-horrors that tell us about Consumer-Man and the run-away menagerie of his overstimulated mind – much the way David Lynch's movies summarise these dark forces in Post-Modern film. *Wild at Heart*, *Blue Velvet*, *Twin Peaks* – these are the equivalents of *Marco Polo*, *Ramesses II* and *Homebase*. Not good (or bad) enough to qualify in this category are many of the Richard Seifert buildings in the Docklands. Fleet House (C3) and *The Daily Telegraph* are marooned in some conceptual swamp between rectitude and glitz. More confections, such as Meridian Gate, Chelsea Harbour and the Saatchi & Saatchi Headquarters, Minster Court and One American Square (C4, C5, C6, C8, C13) are trapped between over-indulgence and sobriety. They never decide whether to enjoy Baroque overstatement and historical reminiscence, or be cheap and thin-skinned. In this they are the perfect expression of yuppie contradiction, Thatcher's Britain, the unacceptable face of rip-off architecture. Puritanical critics, naturally being fascinated by this unforgivable form of sin, call it forth whenever they want to censure Post-Modernism *en bloc*, whereas much of the public will defend it as slightly better than Modernist totalitarian architecture. Was Mussolini better than Hitler? The argument is a stand-off.

However, with the Post-Modernisation of failed or crumbling Modernist buildings, one can now get closer to an answer: a direct comparison is possible. Howell, Killick, Partridge and Amis' Weston Rise Housing Estate in Islington, 1965, was a muscular version of Brutalist push-pull with the main visual problem of being too dark, too grey and too homogeneous (C18). In 1988 the local Council renovated and repainted this urbanism giving the Modernist grammar a kind of Robert Adam articulation. This creates an extraordinarily lively rhythm: elements now jump around, syncopate and vibrate as they never did before. The lightness of tone is pure gain. No wonder vast stretches of Modern concrete housing, from London to Glasgow, are being Post-Modernised – when they are not being blown apart. It's a fate better than death, at least for the cost-conscious Council. Here the five massive blocks snake around a triangular site *à la Smithson* 1963, having the virtue of being made in discrete sections (and so grammatical), yet with the vice of creating leaky, left-over space everywhere. A true Post-Modernisation would have contained these areas, added grass and mixed uses.

Commercial offices, whose concrete is spalling, can also be given a second life. 'Vantage West' used to be one of the deadliest slob blocks (brother of *slab*) one could find on the way in from Heathrow, at the crucial bend in the flyover of the M4 (C19). Now the stacked coffins of horizontal floors are hidden behind a vertical facade of cheery blue glass and flush aluminium. The thin, stilted arches have negative keystones, two left-over cleaning cradles (which are actually called permanent balconies on the drawings). As ornament the facade is a joke, and not very funny, but it does refresh a previously moribund interior and born-dead exterior: it also provides acoustic insulation from the 'roar of famished motor-cars beneath'. In many such cases then, kitsch Post-Modernism is a marginal improvement on the previous mode of building – nothing to cheer about but still less bad.

To recognise this is to remember that architectural judgement is related to two quite different axes of measurement, or varying standards of taste: buildings from the era which has just preceded and the entire history of architecture. Everyone keeps both models somewhere in their mind, even if not very consciously. Judged by these different canons, commercial Post-Modernism is clearly both progressive and regressive. It is functionally more

developed, popular and urbane than commercial Modernism, while it is less adept, gracious and sophisticated than commercial Victorian building.

For instance, if Stirling's Number One Poultry were to be built it would equal the quality of Waterhouse's Manchester Town Hall – an equivalent triangular piece of urbanism in planning and architectural drama. It would not, however, approach this Neo-Gothic structure in terms of ornament and developed iconography. Such mixed architectural judgements are natural today, and they keep one slightly sceptical and alert to complex conclusions. Even with this ambiguity and divergence in mind, however, I admit to being unsure of placing such monoliths as Beaufort House in the City (C21), or Southwark Bridge Offices and Housing (C24). The former is what Stuart Lipton calls 'rent-slab' Post-Modern Classicism – Michael Graves and KPF applied to the formula of maximum return on square footage. It is better urbanistically than its Modernist equivalent, but in 1989 that no longer justifies such stereotypical work. The same is true of the sectioned block that steps up and back next to the Thames – a clear homage to Cascades down the river. It is better than the faceless Modern slabs which disfigure the view from the Tate Gallery, but, in 1990, so what?

Can worse architecture of 30 years ago, in the same commercial genre, legitimise such mediocrities? For the youth and Neo-Modernists it's a clear 'no', for the developer and public it's an ambiguous 'maybe', and for the designer and client it's a hesitant 'yes'. However, time has moved the goal-posts, and what was a step forward for Post-Modernism in 1980 is now, at best, a marching in place since the rest of society has caught up.

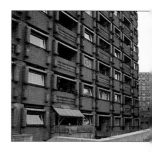

Notting Hill Annual Carnival, 1990.

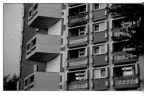

Before and After: Post-Modernisation by paint of HKPA Weston Rise Housing (C18) – the transformation should have gone further.

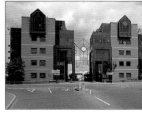

Boom-Bust architecture, Frontier-Docklands architecture, Thatcher architecture, Toy-Town architecture – Rip-off, Yuppie, Dallas, Pastiche, Ghost-town – all the labels have been applied to decorated sheds such as SSC Consultants' Meridian Gate (C4).

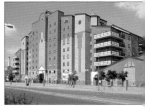

Mixed verdict must be given on much commercial Post-Modernism. Progressive with respect to 60s slab block housing and offices, it is sometimes equal to 19th-century versions of the genre – John Gills' Elm Quay (C24).

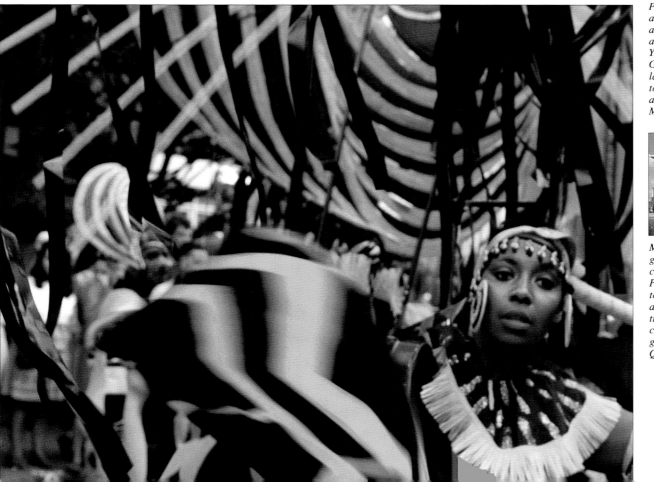

25 CARNIVALESQUE BUILDINGS

C1 *IAN POLLARD, Sainsbury's Homebase, Warwick Road and Fenelon Place W14, 1988. The most sincerely hated building in London is better than one might think. A flat decorated shed building with Egyptian figures and columns mixes High-Tech and Stirling's Stuttgart at crucially visible points. The zig-zags indicate a cut from one style to the next like signs on an architectural drawing. Egyptian gods, taken from British Museum studies, hold various equipment on sale within – including a power drill.*

C2 *IAN POLLARD, Marco Polo House, Queenstown Road SW8, 1986-87. A very curious mélange, this building is one part Modern horizontal office and one part vertical palace, as if Mies van der Rohe married John Vanbrugh and had the offspring kitted out in a new synthetic of stone-glass. Indeed note this shiney white and grey material, it's a form of superstone with the glistening qualities of a rubber-suit. The broken pediment is from Philip Johnson's AT&T, but it's more wild here; the blank, elephantine scale of the legs, wall and top relate to the huge gasometer and Battersea Power station nearby. All in all a Pop-Classical response to the surrounding road context with the added surprise of a High-Tech and comfortable interior. The Observer journalists are said to like the whole building – even Stephen Gardiner!*

C3 *RICHARD SEIFERT LTD, Fleet House, Marsh Wall, Docklands E14, 1988-89. These offices are the kind of building high-minded Modernist critics love to hate as 'toy-town' architecture because the forms have the sophistication of a four-year old's building blocks. But there is an irony here. When Frank Lloyd Wright used the Froebel Block method of composing buildings it was fresh, inventive and productive of an open system of building, whereas here Classical 'blocks' produce the old closed Renaissance aesthetic with full corner stops marked in grey granite and all the volumes edged by surrounding ornament. Wright placed his grey ornamental bands at right angles to the volumes and thus set up a counterpoint; here they reinforce each other. Well, the results are obvious, clunky, flat and diagrammatic, but paradoxically all of this is quite new in feeling. The building is as fresh as an* ingenue. *It looks as if Seifert had decided to 'do' Brunelleschi on the computer and build the Early Renaissance two inches thick, and flat. That's new and curious. Note the strange indented corners and absent cornice and the way the conceptual grey 'frame' is out of synch with the real structure and windows: odd.*

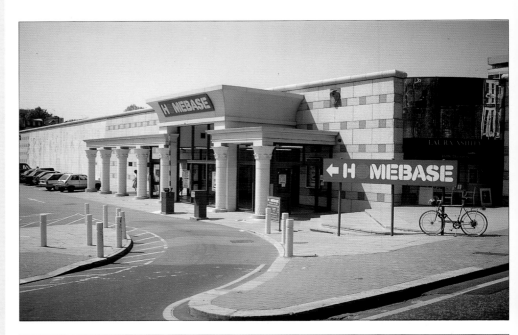

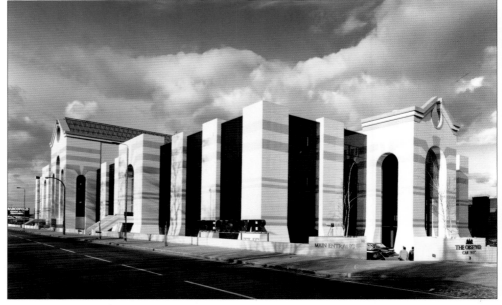

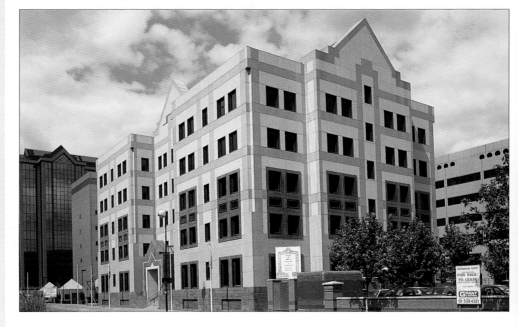

C4 *SSC CONSULTANTS LTD, Meridian Gate, Marsh Wall, Docklands E14, 1988- (three phases, the first complete 1990). This is Frontier Architecture of the Docklands with the unmistakable air of the boom and bust about it. Toy-town and High-Tech at the front while Bloated Pedimental at the back – the elephantine red pediments really have to be seen to be believed.*

C5 *RAY MOXLEY (MOXLEY, LENNER AND PARTNERS), Chelsea Harbour SW10, 1986- 89. '36 retail units, 95 studios and offices, 310 residential units (18 houses) 75-berth marina, 160-suite hotel, five restaurants. Fancy prices'. The architecture is interesting as a compilation of clichés – particularly the High-Tech aluminium tower with its pagodoid roof and golden bauble, or its Robert Adam town-houses mixed with Mediterranean marina; but in the end the sociology of this Yuppie haven is more interesting.*

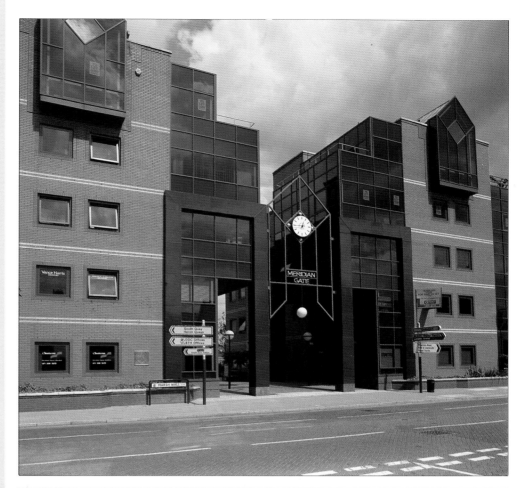

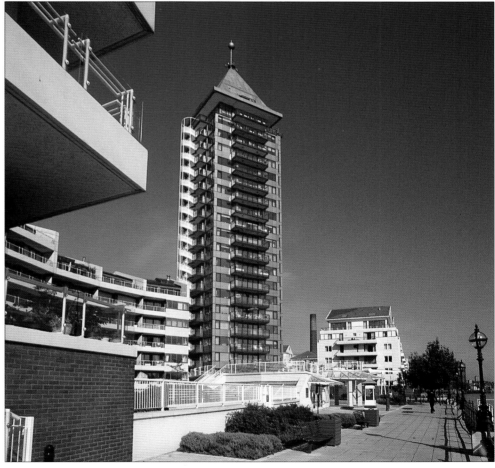

C6 CHAPMAN TAYLOR, Lansdowne House, Berkeley Square W1, 1987-88. The typical groundscraper, but reduced to the scale of Mayfair, it has the ubiquitous grand atrium carefully overseen by security guards. While Modernists sneer it down as Dallas glitz and bash the size of its LA Door, I find its ground floor layering one of the more interesting moves in Post-Modern articulation. The fractured planes are almost Cubist, the ornamental incisions both fresh and well-scaled, the mixture of greys and blues, polished and rough stone, very convincing. If only the whole building had attained this Free-Style inventiveness.

C7 CHAPMAN TAYLOR, First Interstate House, 14 Agar Street, Strand WC2, 1988. Next to the 1907 Zimbabwe House by Charles Holden, this building rings the changes on similar Mannerist motifs – ABA windows, an attic floor of vertical windows, pier buttresses and arches. Clad in Portland stone these pretentious muscular forms march over a granite plinth of arches and heavy keystones. The flat, shallow layering is the standard Post-Modern device to increase the feeling of depth and accentuate the bones, eyelids and flesh of an essentially plain office.

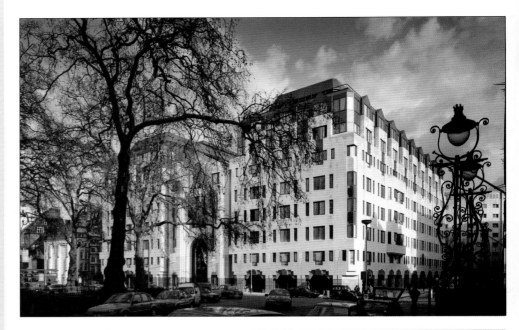

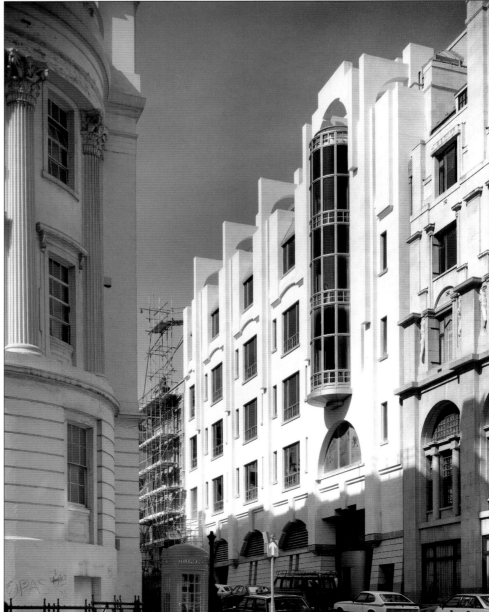

C8 *GMW PARTNERSHIP, Minster Court, Mincing Lane and Mark Lane EC3, 1988-91. Three blocks of office, retailing and restaurant for Prudential, this scheme has one of the spookiest roofscapes since the Witches House was built in Los Angeles. Peeked pitches jostle about the site like a coven of shrouded hags – no question the image is intentional even if no one can explain it. The facades are clad in pink/grey Torcicoda granite with flamed and polished finishes, but it is really the blank windows and almost Cubist facets which make this building nicely haunting. Perhaps this was an accident?*

C9 *CASSON CONDOR, Ismaili Centre, Thurloe Place SW7, 1980-83. Moghul top, Mackintoshian bottom and thin-windowed middle with the volumes accentuated by a blue line. Conceptually this is a geode with a hard masonry revealing a soft, iridescent underbelly; the main problems are the heavy massing and truncated gestures.*

C10 *REOVEN VARDI, Lycée Français Charles de Gaulle, Harrington Road and Queensberry Way SW7, 1982. Conceptually this is a fine rhythmical bay solution which recalls Mackintosh's Glasgow School of Art in elevation and some details, but the construction lets the scheme down. As a drawing or model the forms would have had more integration and one wouldn't be so put off by the white bathroom tiles and clunky glazing. Still, this is a sympathetic urban infill and comment on the previous Lycée.*

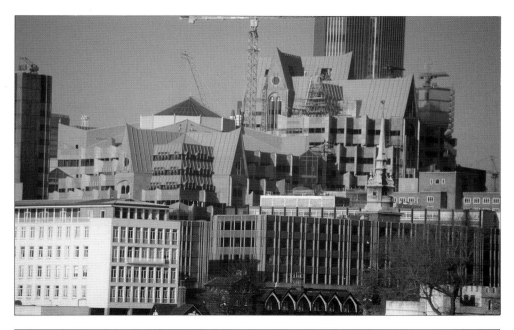

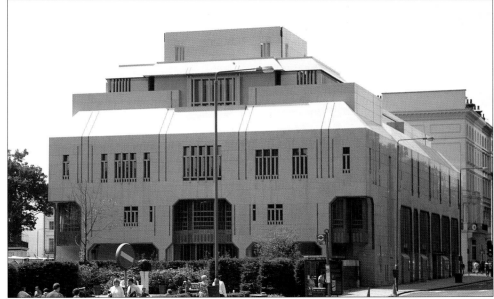

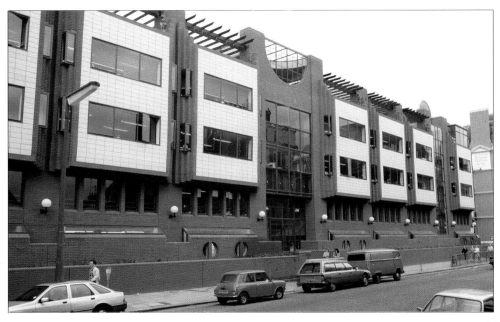

C11 *RENTON HOWARD WOOD LEVIN, 20 Old Bailey EC4, 1989. Post-Modern Classicism at its worst, this is the most ungrammatical, diagrammatical pastiche in the City which somehow – bad as it is – even manages to avoid the final redemption of being 'so bad that it's good'.*

C12 *DAMOND LOCK GRABOWSKI & PARTNERS, St George's House, 6 Eastcheap EC3, 1989-90. Post-Modern Classicism woven together with different coloured polished masonry. Note how the bay window breaks through the cornice level leaving the trace of a flare and then re-emerges with a cap and keystone. The Free-Style may be naïve, but it has an undeniable vitality. (Same architects as B28)*

C13 *RENTON HOWARD WOOD LEVIN PARTNERSHIP, One America Square, Crosswall & Fenchurch Street Station EC3, 1989-91. Multi-occupancy office, 200-feet and 15-storeys tall, the Art-Deco Classicism has been attacked by Modernists for being 'paper-thin architecture' – 'wallpaper' applied to a steel frame, only two-inches thick. But of course that was the point of the 'free facade' according to Modernists. For Le Corbusier the curtain wall allowed the facade to follow the architect's chosen laws of composition: the fact that here these are Free-Style Classicism may be objectionable to people with a prejudice against this style and iconography, but it only shows that they have failed to understand their own Modernist injunctions of freedom. The vertical massing counteracts the horizontality of the block, while the 'Jencksiana' emphasises the front door and long faces of the side elevations and the colours and mouldings break down the volume. The result is far superior to the architects' Beaufort House (C21) from which it stems.*

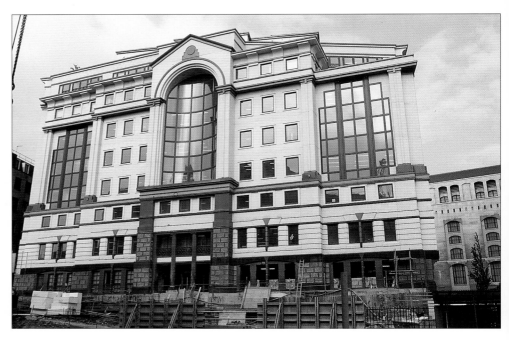

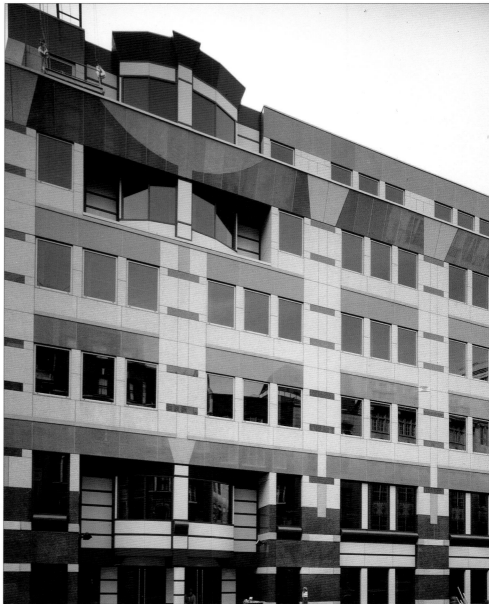

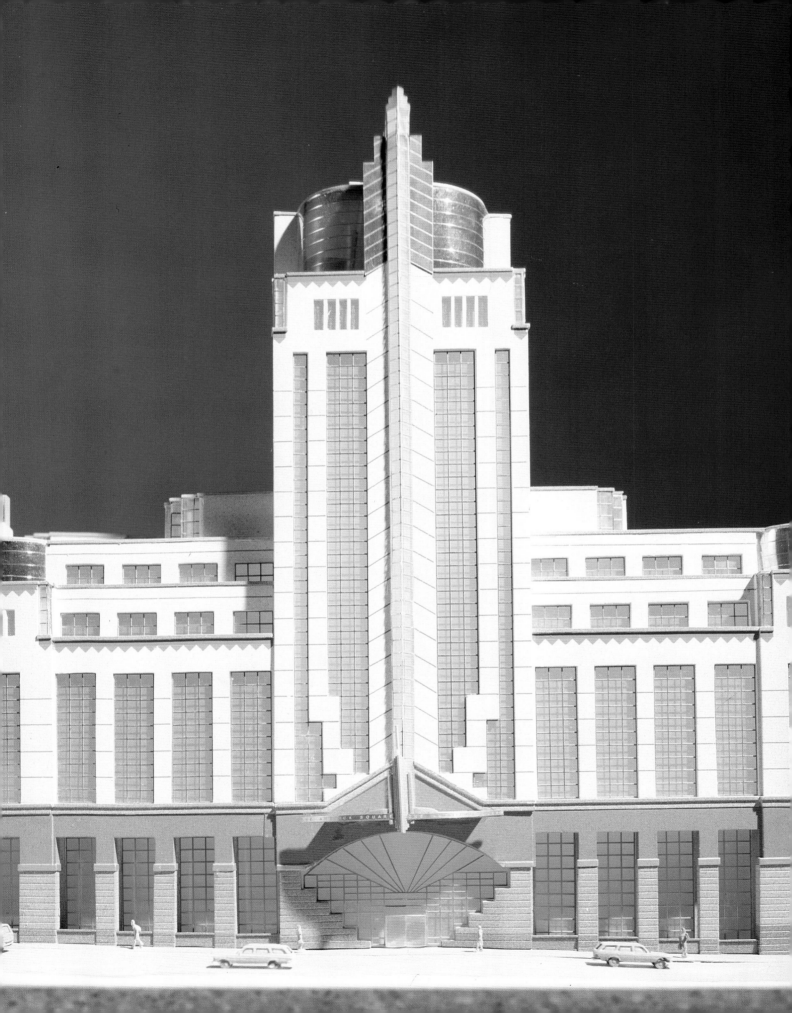

C14 ARCHITECH (now known as COM-PREHENSIVE DESIGN GROUP), Admiral House, 60-66 East Smithfield (corner Dock Street) E1, 1987-88. This is a naïve but exuberant collage of Post-Modern elements enjoyed for their insubstantiality. The ubiquitous V-forms, triangles in green, and prow-like balconies (Dock Street) are played against wrapping pediments and framing downspouts. The fun of the game can be seen in the horizontal and vertical windows which fight it out, and the different materials and forms which are layered tightly on top of each other. At first one is reminded of Leopold Eidelitz's despairing definition of American architecture: 'The art of covering one thing with another thing to resemble a third thing which, even if it were original, would not be desirable'. But here there is no attempt to counterfeit – only half clothe (or is it half reveal?).

C15 ELSOM PACK & ROBERTS, 90 Fenchurch Street EC3, 1989-90. This seven-storey Post-Modern Classical office is symmetrical around its large central door and full of internal symmetries. Gentle semicircles protrude hesitantly in a central bay window and top pediment, while cream and grey stone and black and white windows play games of hide-and-seek across the facade. This gives it more interest than the neighbours it respects.

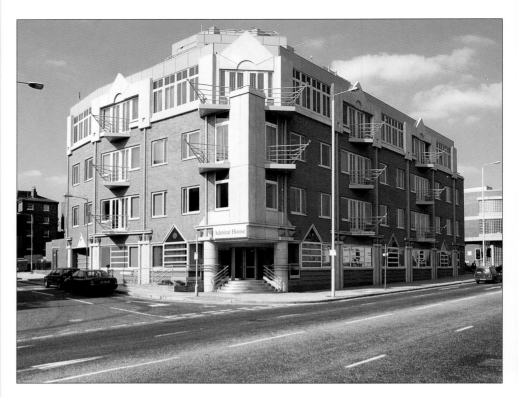

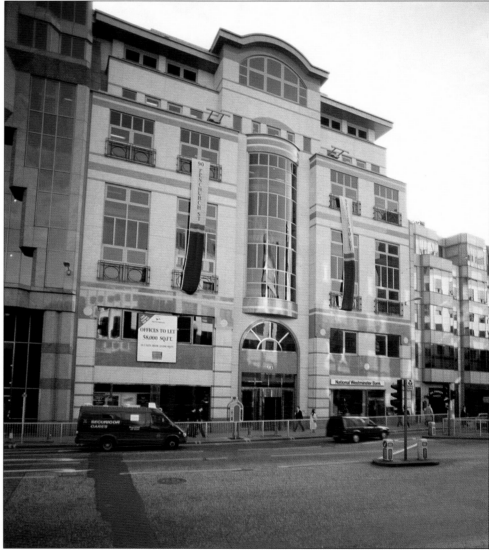

C16 ELSWORTH SYKES PARTNERSHIP, *Strand Bridge House, 138-142 The Strand WC2, 1989. Lugubrious Second Empire Mansardic with neutron-bomb finials, toy-town window surrounds and an awkward dumpiness that is endearing. This is failed pretentiousness at its best.*

C17 FITZROY ROBINSON, *Drury House, Drury Lane and Russell Street WC2, 1988-89. Glitzy pink, green and orange palazzo with industrial cornice and corner cylinders – the combination which used to be known as 'industrial Classicism' when applied to the Michelin House in 1907, here has the vulgarity but not the panache of its predecessor.*

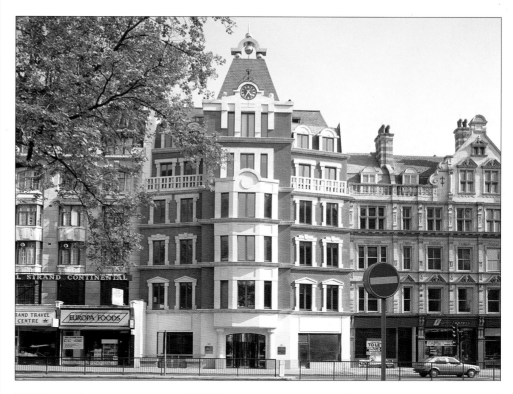

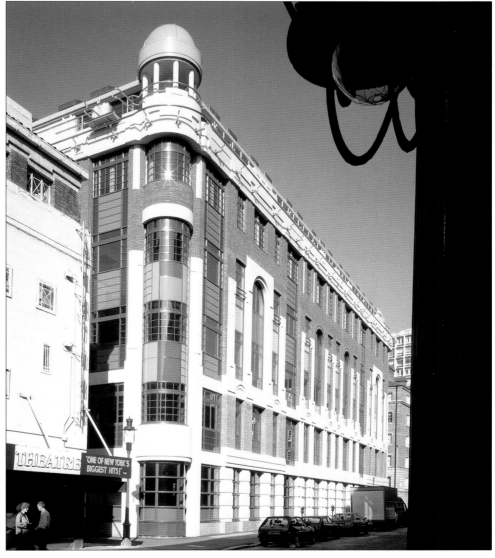

C18 *HOWELL, KILLICK, PARTRIDGE & AMIS, Weston Rise Housing Estate, Islington N1, 1965; refurbished 1988. Brutalist slab blocks tilted to each other and snaking around an urban site – destroying the opportunity of any contained space – have been transformed into a lighter more dynamic and syncopated architecture by the polychromy. If only this Post-Modernisation were extended to the space and function.*

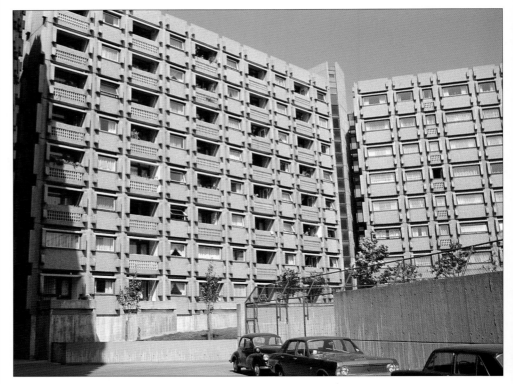

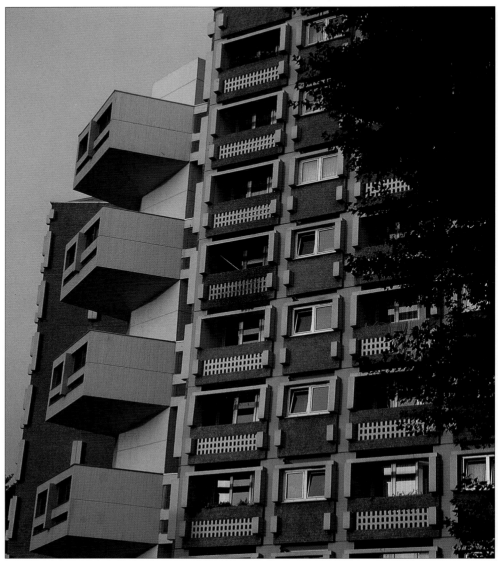

C19 *COVELL MATTHEWS WHEATLEY,*
Vantage West, M4 Motorway at Hammer-
smith W6, 1965 and refurbished 1989. The
refacing and transformation of the 60s slab
block in cheery blue glass, flush joints and
high, stilted arches. The balconies are not,
as they look, cleaning cranes. However much
one may criticise this pastiche, it is superior
to the Modernist block it transforms – visu-
ally, environmentally and acoustically for
the users.

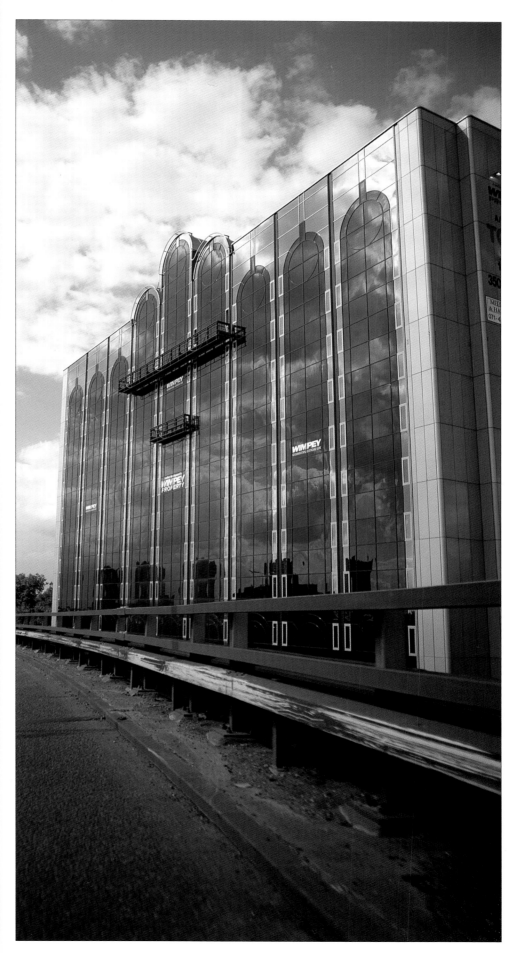

C20 SHEPPARD ROBSON, *338 Euston Road NW1, offices, 1990. This office refit is a clear improvement on the original Modern slab block of the 1960s. The two long sides have been extended 1.5 metres as can be seen by the attractive Z-shaped structural members that run up the front and back. An ultra cool Free-Style Classicism orders the facades – grey steel versus black tinted solar glass – in a regular rhythm of seven bays on the west side, while the front has a pleasant, semicircular bay window that culminates in a 16th-floor balcony, and curved mouldings. The most interesting aspect is the Post-Modern columnar order – air-conditioning risers which are given storey high 'absent' capitals – and a dignified presence. These resulted because the cramped 60s office had little room for the ducts: necessity was here the mother of Post-Modern Classicism.*

C21 RENTON HOWARD WOOD LEVIN, *Beaufort House, Petticoat Lane and Aldgate Roundabout E1, 1986-88. Rent-slab Post-Modern Classicism on the American model of KPF and Michael Graves. The scale is inevitably bloated and High Imperial Roman with a six-storey entrance and heavy broken pediment in ruddy brown marble. Polished and smooth granite, rustications, banded courses, setbacks, mouldings – all the Classical paraphernalia are applied to make this monolith less monolithic. Financial motives were uppermost, but Mammon, it has to be said, would be far uglier and massive without the articulations.*

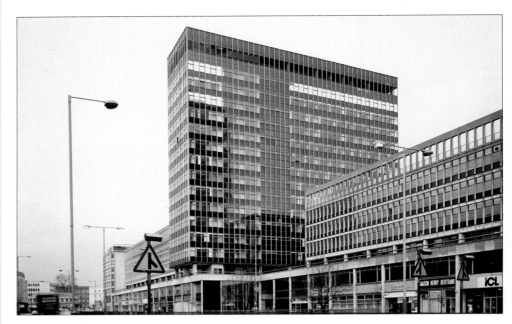

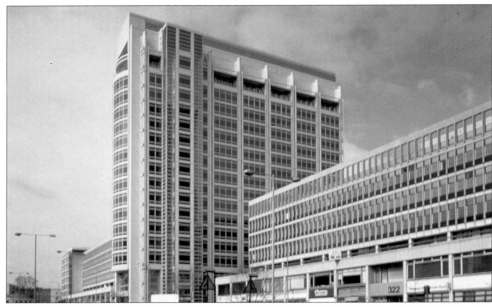

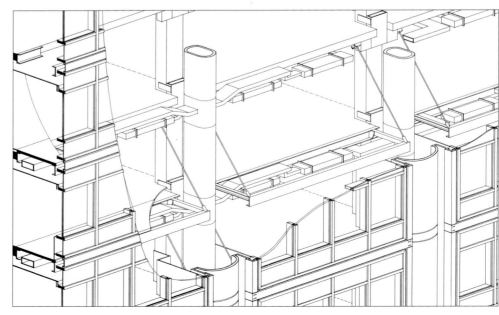

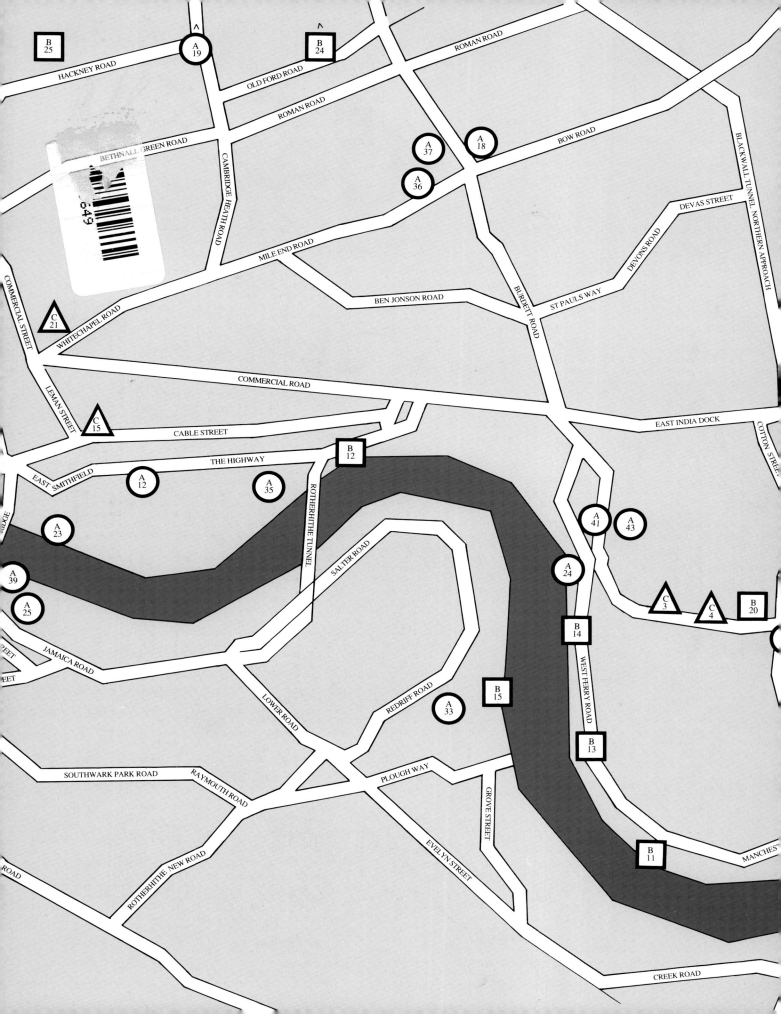

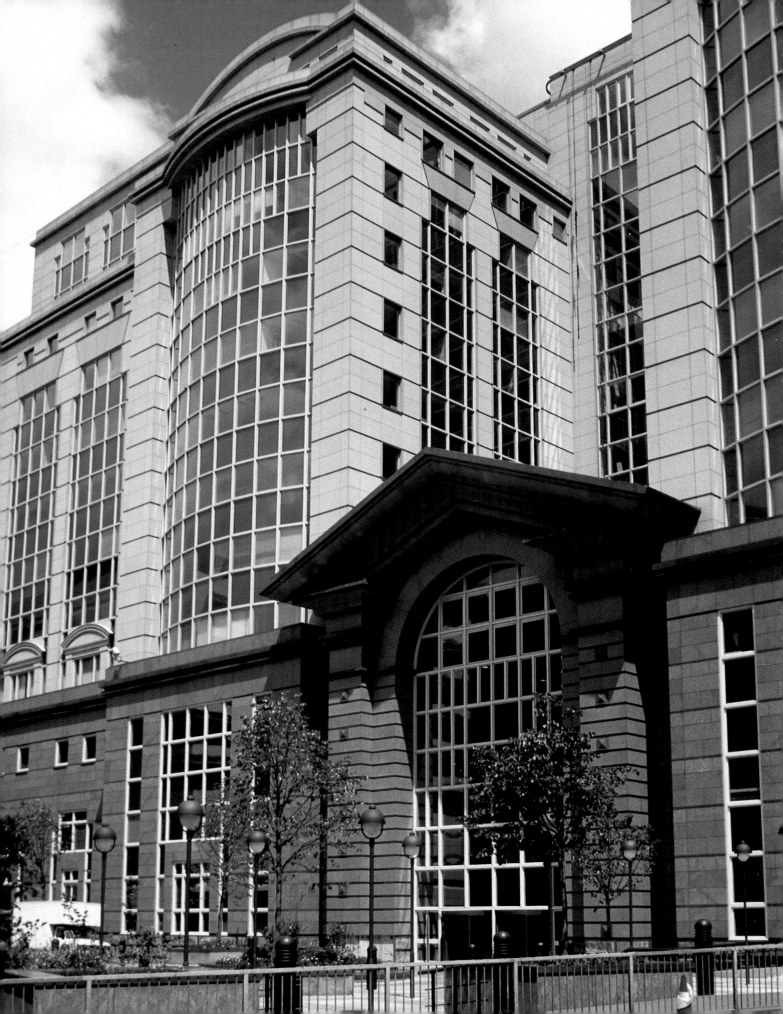

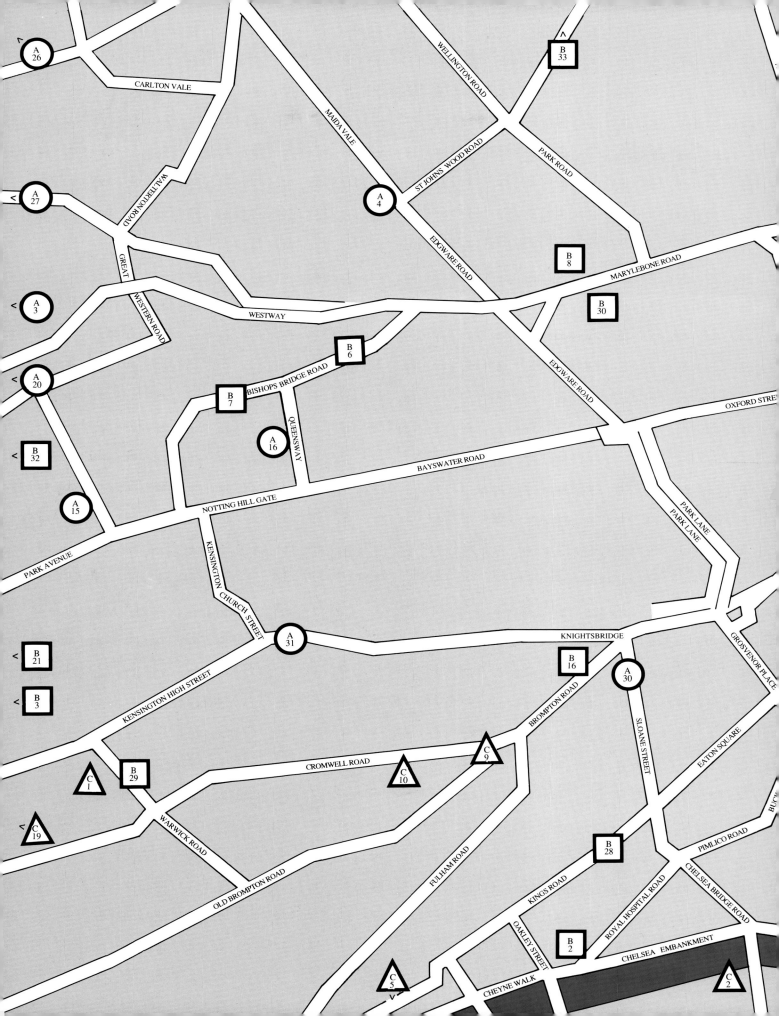

C24 *JOHN GILLS, Elm Quay, 22-30 Nine Elms Lane, SW8, 1988-89. A 10-storey pyramidal slab block of offices and housing is broken up, on the street side, into nine vertical bays to lessen the horizontal dimension. Further articulations of brick colour and pattern – and white balconies – cut up the bulk. On the river side a giant broken pediment weaves through the vertical brick rectangles and pulls together the triangular elements.*

C25 *ARCHITECH, Michael House, 35 Chiswell Street EC1, 1989-90. Another pastiche from those who brought you Admiral House (C15), it is better than its dumpy volume and clunky details at first suggest. The step-down logic of the attic floors, the way the street line is held and the main entrance and service entrance are marked, make a lot of sense. The bull nose sills, staccato ornament and flat mouldings even have the logic of the blank glazing – all very direct.*

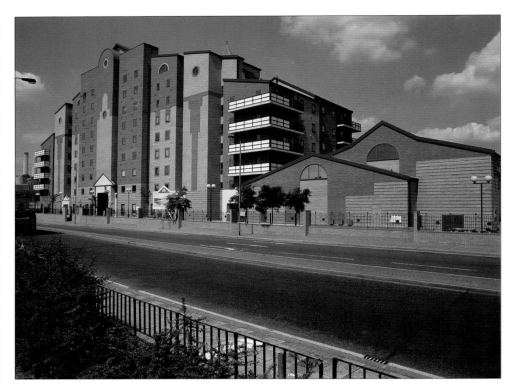

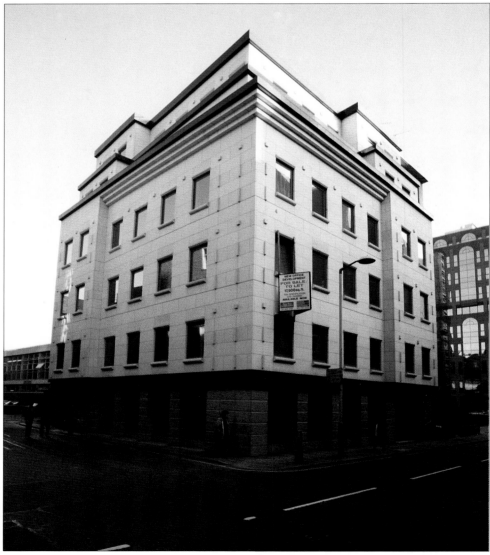

C22 *CECIL DENNY & HIGHTON, Tower Bridge Court, Tower Bridge and Horselydown Lane SE1, 1988-91. Street-smart architecture filling a block, holding the street lines and, in Horselydown Lane, making something interesting out of a rhythmical bay system which has an equal emphasis on brick, cast stone and glass. The ubiquitous V-shaped windows, flared 'Ionic' capitals and ultra-thin cornice are worth remarking. On the Tower Bridge side, Post-Modern motifs abound including a Stirlingesque curve, 'Jencksiana' scuppers, and Free-Style Classical details. Thus another urbane chameleon changing its spots, but in search of an environment in which to fit.*

C23 *ROLFE JUDD GROUP, Barclays Bank & Offices, Soho Square W1, 1987-88. Layered with stone echelons and dripping with balls of all sorts, this corner building, with its split pediment, is not a bad urban hinge between a lower street and a high-storeyed square. The grammar combines Art Deco and the Wrennaissance of brick and white trim.*

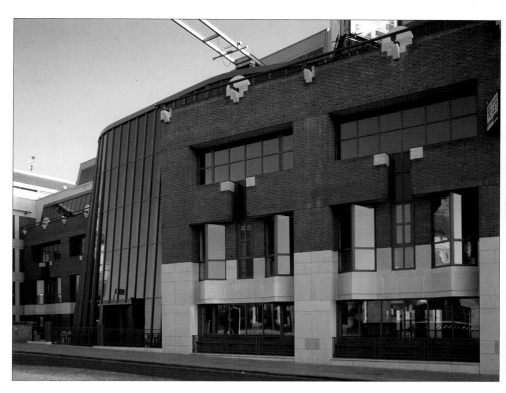

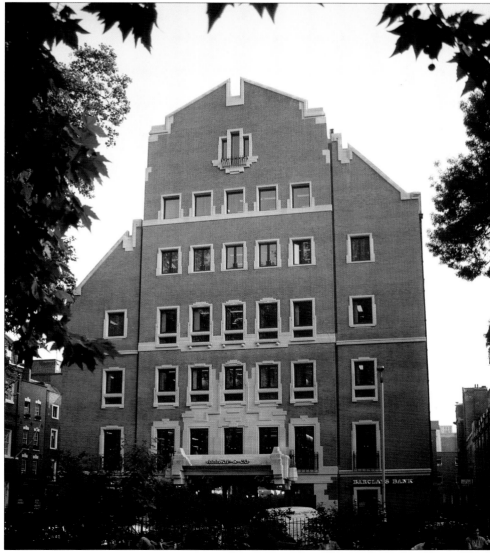

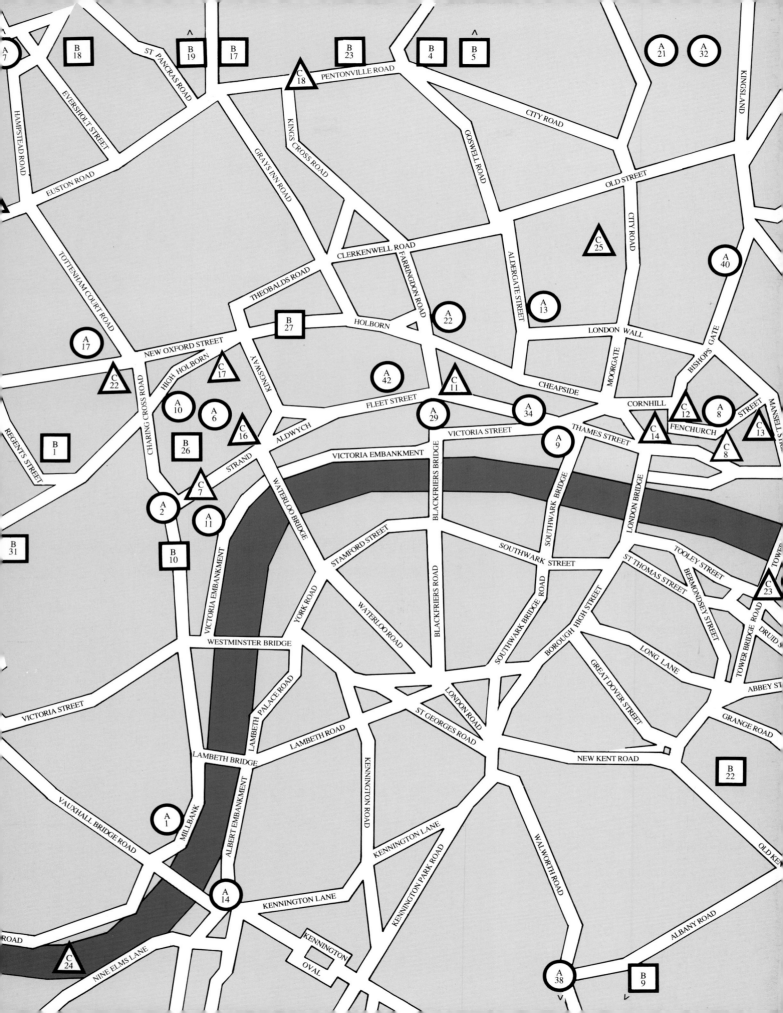